Weights
for **Weight Loss**

Weights

for Weight Loss

Fat-Burning and
Muscle-Sculpting Exercises
with over 200 Step-by-Step Photos

ELLEN BARRETT

photography by Robert Holmes

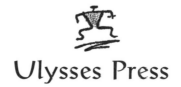

Ulysses Press

Published in the United States by
Ulysses Press
P.O. Box 3440
Berkeley, CA 94703
www.ulyssespress.com

ISBN 1-56975-514-0
Library of Congress Control Number 2005930014

Printed in Canada by Webcom Limited

10 9 8 7 6 5 4 3 2 1

Editorial/Production	Lily Chou, Claire Chun, Nicholas Denton-Brown, Matt Orendorff, Steven Zah Schwartz, Kathryn Brooks
Cover design	Leslie Henriques
Photography	Robert Holmes, except photograph on page 20 © photos.com
Model	Ellen Barrett

Clothing provided by Capezio

Distributed by Publishers Group West

Please Note
This book has been written and published strictly for informational purposes, and in no way should be used as a substitute for consultation with health care professionals. You should not consider educational material herein to be the practice of medicine or to replace consultation with a physician or other medical practitioner. The author and publisher are providing you with information in this work so that you can have the knowledge and can choose, at your own risk, to act on that knowledge. The author and publisher also urge all readers to be aware of their health status and to consult health care professionals before beginning any health program.

contents

part one:

getting started

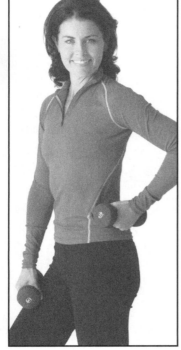

introduction

Want to lose weight, look better and feel energized? You've picked up the right book! *Weights for Weight Loss* is about losing weight *properly* and keeping it off *easily*. If you're one of the millions of people who yo-yo up and down on the scale, going on and off of diets, this program presents something different. You won't find any speeches here about reducing calories. Rather, this is a modern manual that will show you how to increase your energy output using handheld weights, resulting in weight loss without deprivation.

Throughout my nearly 20 years in the fitness industry, I've witnessed a lot of workout trends, like aerobics, Jazzercise, step aerobics, *tae bo*, yoga and Pilates. And I've seen many diet trends, too, like the grapefruit, the Zone, the Atkins and the South Beach diets. These fads tend to debut with a bang and seem instantly to become part of popular culture. People talk about them at dinner parties and around the water cooler. They're featured on the covers of *Time* magazine and *Newsweek*. They achieve Super Bowl status in popularity. Then, the tide begins to turn and the spotlight starts to dim. America seems to telepathically shout, "On to the next one!"

My reason for writing this is not to discredit other workout and weight-loss techniques. They have all proven effective for some part of the population at some point in time. Someone, somewhere, has found health, wellness and weight-loss success with each of these trends, and that's truly a triumph. We all understand that weight loss isn't easy! Millions of people struggle to lose weight all their lives, and meet with failure again and again. If one of these trends helps even just one person, it deserves a round of applause.

My purpose in mentioning these fad diets and workout trends is to frame an important point about this book. Weight training has never been a hot trend. It has never been "all the rage." It's not front-page news. But it has always been here. Weight training is a workout *and* weight-loss technique that has withstood the test of time. Working out with weights (not to be mistaken for the sport of body building, which debuted in 12th-century India) was around before aerobics and the grapefruit diet, and it's still here. In fact, it hasn't even ebbed or flowed in popularity. It's been a consistent part of the fitness world since its birth in the late 1970s. For many soundly fit people, weight training has been *and is* a true-blue staple. It's refreshing to know that, throughout my entire career, one thing hasn't changed.

I suspect that there are three core reasons for this. First, weight training works for men and women, for all ages, and for every fitness level. Few fitness workouts are so inclusive. Second, weight training offers many variants, so there's less risk of ending up in the "workout rut." One can adjust the size of the weight, the angle of the movement, the range of motion and even the sequence of exercises. The countless number of viable routines makes for constant mental engagement and physical challenge. Third, weight training is the epitome of "low maintenance." There is no need for large spaces, special clothing, a specific location or big bucks. Weight training is practical, accommodating and cheap. And what great news! Weight training is our user-friendly ticket to lasting weight loss.

The Weight Loss Prerequisite

Before you begin to play the weight-loss game, the one and only prerequisite is simply to make up your mind to take charge of your weight. And because there are two big, controllable variables in the weight-loss game—the amount of calories you take in and the amount of calories you burn—taking charge is easier than you may think. Even though it may not appear so at times, you are very much in control of those numbers on the bathroom scale. From now on, your DNA, your sedentary job and your inability to afford a trainer three times per week are not to be blamed for any weight woes. Explaining this way of thinking to my training clients is a highlight for me because it's truly empowering. "You're the C.E.O of Y.O.U.," I've been known to exclaim with conviction. The first step is realizing that the ball is in your court when it comes to losing weight and keeping it off. Your thoughts and actions dictate the outcome. That's why the first exercise in this book isn't a bicep curl, it's a straightforward mental move: You must take responsibility for your weight. It's as easy as making up your mind to do so.

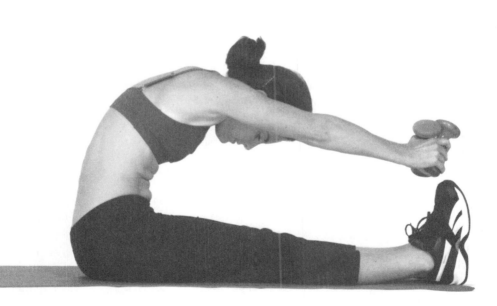

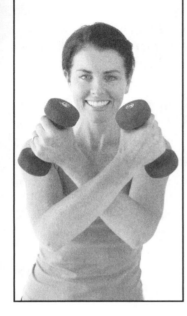

the ABCs of weight loss

The formula for losing weight is actually very simple: Consume less energy than you burn. The way we tend to measure food energy in the body is by counting calories. Just as watts measure electrical energy in a light bulb, calories measure heat energy in the body. I personally don't focus on calories in my everyday life, and I encourage my clients to avoid caloric obsession.

However, for the purpose of this mini science lesson, we must focus on this simple fact: The one and only scientifically proven method for losing weight involves burning more calories than the amount consumed.

Thus, it follows that there are two ways to lose weight. You can reduce your caloric intake or increase your metabolic rate. Eat less, burn more! On paper, the act of losing weight doesn't seem so difficult, does it? But if it's such a cinch, then why do millions of people carry excess weight, or lose it only to gain it all back and then some? To answer this question, let's look at the concept of metabolism.

Metabolism

People tend to make the concept of metabolism one-dimensional, thinking it's related merely to the intake and use of food. When a person is thin, we generalize and say, "Oh, they've been blessed with a fast metabolism." When someone struggles with their weight, they may complain, "I have a sluggish metabolism." While all of this may be true, it's not the whole story. Metabolism has three major components that are advantageous to recognize.

Basal Metabolism Rate: Also known as the *resting metabolic rate*, the basal metabolism is the energy used when the body is at complete rest. It involves

the calories used to keep all systems going day in and day out—the calories burned by the brain, heart, kidneys and all organs and cells in the body. About two-thirds to three-quarters of the calories we burn everyday are accounted for in basal metabolism. The basal metabolism is closely related to one's muscle mass, so we actually have a bit of control over our basal metabolism in that we can increase our own muscle mass.

Active Metabolism Rate: This second component of metabolism is the calories burned in activities such as walking, stair climbing, picking up children, and dedicated exercise. It corresponds to one's

CALORIES

A calorie (technically called kilocalories or kcal) by definition is the amount of heat required to raise one kilogram of water one degree centigrade. Calories are the units of measurement that the western world uses to quantify the fuel energy that is available from food and to measure the heat output that comes from metabolism, which is the number of calories the body burns.

activity level. Calories burned in physical activity are the most variable part of metabolism—this is the component over which we have the most control. Active metabolism can account for approximately 30 percent of our energy usage.

Digestive Metabolism Rate: This third component is the caloric output used to digest and absorb food. A relatively small percentage of calories—about 10 percent—are burned to digest and absorb food. Basically, eating calories uses calories.

In sum, we burn calories three ways: by being alive and having physical bodies, by moving our bodies and by feeding our bodies. This important information helps us to understand the mechanics of the human body when it comes to weight loss. If you thought that when it came to weight loss the cards were stacked against you, think again. You're actually a calorie-burning machine. If you're alive, you're burning calories. Weight training can increase the basal metabolic rate and the active metabolic rate, making it doubly effective for weight loss.

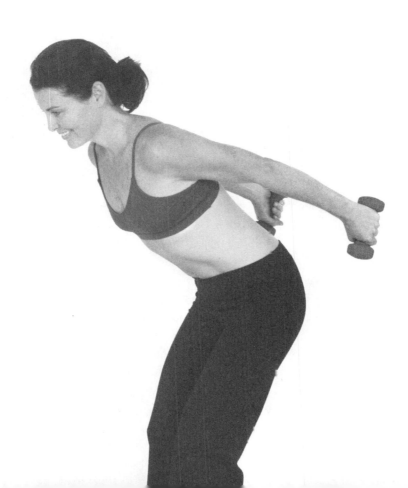

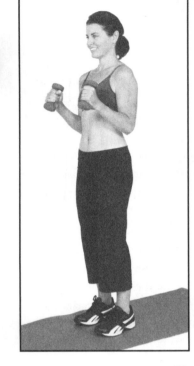

a balanced body

A healthy body is a balanced body. Everything matters, and everything is connected. This means that how you eat, sleep and live your life aside from your 10-, 20-, 30- or 40-minute weight-training routine influences weight-loss success. You'll notice that there's a reccurring theme in this section: balance.

Weights for Weight Loss focuses on the workout side of losing weight, but the dietary aspect of losing weight plays an enormous role, which I feel I must touch on to make this book complete. In conjunction with increased calorie burn, to lose weight you may have to reduce your caloric intake, too. This *must* be done in a balanced manner, however—nothing too drastic. Skipping meals, avoiding carbohydrates, and fasting are three unhealthy ways to attempt weight loss. Very low-calorie diets do not work. Fat-free diets do not work. No-carb diets do not work. They're all extreme and unbalanced, and though they may initially result in weight loss, permanent weight loss will remain

elusive. "Stay away from anything extreme" is another one of my big mottos. Extremes in eating throw the body way out of whack and wreak havoc on our total health, not just our waistlines.

Much is written on diet and dieting, as you probably know. Every day we are barraged with food messages from the media, health professionals and well-intentioned acquaintances. The implied promises from infomercials and diet drugs—they make me dizzy! We label food "good" or "bad" one day, then turn around to find what was "bad" is suddenly our ticket to slim. Because of this insane mix of messages, it's unfortunately completely normal to be confused about eating. How

much should we eat? When? What? How often? The answer to all these questions, in one word, is *balance*.

Balanced Eating Strategies

A balanced diet contains carbohydrates, protein, fat, vitamins, mineral salts, and fiber. It contains these things in the correct proportions. Each body has its own individual needs, but there are some general guidelines that are helpful to all.

- Eat a wide variety of food from all food groups.
- Have less food at each meal but increase the number of nutritious meals or snacks per day.
- Reduce your intake of foods that are low in

nutrients (i.e., "empty calories"), like soda and candy. Some energy-dense foods that are high in nutrients (such as red meat, nuts, avocados, extra-virgin olive oil) can be included in small amounts.

- Cut down on saturated fats.
- Reduce alcohol consumption.
- Try to eat more fresh foods and fewer processed foods.
- Avoid using food for comfort, such as when you are upset, angry or stressed.
- Try to stop eating once you feel full.

I know scores of women who have been "on a diet" for so long that they don't know how to be balanced with their eating; I call them "diet-aholics." Their eating patterns have become terribly erratic and they are trapped in a never-ending lose/gain cycle. If you find your eating habits spinning out of control, I suggest you consult a dietitian. Your health insurance may even cover this cost, but even if it doesn't, investing in dietary help is absolutely worth it if it can get you off the diet roller coaster once and for all. Many people spend hundreds of dollars every week on a personal trainer, but very few pay to see a nutritionist.

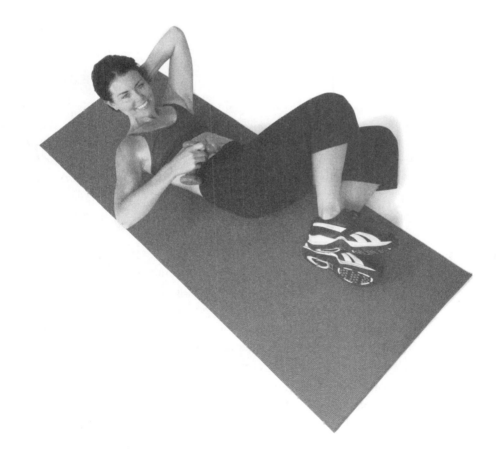

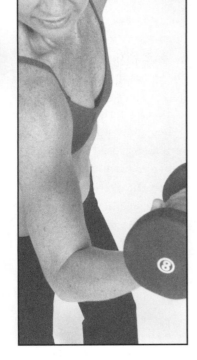

weights for weight loss

Weight training is resistance exercise. The goal is to maintain or increase muscle mass and tone. It's a way to develop muscle strength and create definition throughout the entire body. Whereas body building and weight *lifting* are competitive sports, weight training is not. It's simply a great way to condition the body.

People wonder, seeing as there are seemingly so many ways to lose weight, why I think weight training is the way to go. My answer: Weight training has been scientifically proven to help people lose weight *and keep it off*. In my opinion, losing weight and then regaining it is worse than not losing at all. Not only is it taxing on the body, it ruins self-esteem and has been linked to bouts of depression. I am an advocate for losing weight and keeping it off forever, which is the genius of weight training. Here are the three reasons why weight training allows for a more permanent weight loss:

1. During Effect. Weight training increases the heart rate, which in turn burns more calories. Yes, we actually are getting a bit of cardio when we weight train! Weight training is physical activity and it gobbles up calories, just like walking or dancing.

2. After Effect. When we build additional muscle mass, the basal metabolic rate burns off more calories, even when we are not engaged in physical activity. Remember, muscle burns more calories than fat. For every extra pound of muscle you put on, your body uses around 50 extra calories a day. This is because muscle is metabolically more active than fat and burns more calories than other body tissue, even when you're not moving. In addition, a pound of muscle takes up three-quarters the space of a pound of fat, so strength training helps you slim down even if you don't lose weight.

3. Maintenance Effect. People who lift weights on a regular basis generally sleep more restfully than people who don't. This matters greatly when it comes to weight loss and/or weight maintenance, because the body repairs and restores itself during sleep. When our bodies are deprived of quality sleep, all nine systems in the body (digestive, nervous, skeletal, cardiovascular, lymphatic, endocrine, nervous, reproductive and urinary) work in a less than optimal state, which results in a sluggish metabolism and erratic hormone levels. A fascinating series of studies published in the *Journal of the American Medical Association* and *The Lancet* (an independent medical journal) shows that sleep loss disrupts a series of complex and interwoven metabolic and hormonal processes. This can make weight loss far more difficult than it needs to be.

Busting Six Weight-Training Myths

It's amazing how pervasive inaccurate beliefs about muscle, fat and body function are. Once and for all, I'm here to give you the facts and nix the fiction.

Myth #1: You Can Spot-Reduce Fat from the Human Body

It's painful to watch some of those TV infomercials that claim you can "lose five inches from your waist with the AbMaster," or statements similar in nature. These assertions are just not true. If they were, the area around our mouths

A study done by the University of Colorado reports that lifting weights will work overtime to make you look leaner. Yes, the obvious benefit is beautiful muscle tone, but there's another one. Women who did four sets of ten exercises that targeted major body parts torched up to 60 extra calories in the hour right after lifting, and continued burning at a higher level the rest of the day.

- Enhanced bone modeling to increase bone strength and reduce the risk of osteoporosis
- Stronger connective tissues to increase joint stability and help prevent injury
- Increased functional strength for sports and daily activity
- Increased lean body mass and decreased body fat
- Higher metabolic rate because of an increase in muscle and a decrease in fat
- Improved self-esteem and confidence

---

would be completely fat-free and sunken in from talking and eating every day of our lives! In the case of the abdominals, training with sit-ups and crunches will serve only to increase muscle tone in that area. Fat is lost throughout the body in a pattern dependent upon one's genetics. (Your genes determine where your body fat is stored.) Overall body fat must be reduced to lose fat in any particular area. In order to lose weight in one spot, you must be willing to work your entire body. That is why each of the workouts in this book is geared toward total body training. The women who want thinner hips and the men who wish to shed the spare tire must attack the body as a whole.

Myth #2: Fat Turns into Muscle

Not true. Muscle is muscle, fat is fat. When you increase your muscle mass, you increase your metabolism, which helps burn off more fat. Fat disappears; it

isn't converted into muscle. A fat cell and a muscle cell are two completely unique entities.

Myth #3: Weight Training Leads to Bulky Muscles

The myth that leads many women to reject weight training is the belief that lifting weights causes big muscles. In reality, women simply do not have enough muscle-building hormones to allow for increased muscle mass. In fact, women have 10 to 30 times less of those essential hormones than men. The extreme bodies that we see in muscle magazines are the result of absolute devotion to the sport of body building, along with a rare genetic disposition for accumulating muscle mass. Weight training for fitness and weight-loss purposes usually makes women look smaller, tighter and more "pulled in."

Myth #4: Weight Training Is Just for Men

Weight training benefits women as well as men and is

an ideal exercise regimen for both sexes. Time and time again, research shows that having good muscle tone helps men and women alike live healthier lives. Women especially should appreciate that strength training increases bone density dramatically, reducing the risk of osteoporosis.

Myth #5: Weight Training Increases the Risk of Injury

Actually, studies show the opposite. An increase in strength of bones, muscles and connective tissue (the tendons and ligaments) decreases the risk of injury. More injuries occur as a result of pure cardio-vascular exercises, such as running, biking and step class.

Myth #6: I Need to Lift Heavy Weights to Make an Impact

Heavy weights are effective, but light weights can be effective, too. It all depends on what you're trying to achieve. For weight loss, both heavy and light weights can work well. What's important is to challenge the muscle, and, for many of us, light weights may just do the trick. A big benefit to light weights is that they allow for bigger range of motion, which feels good and may provide a slight stretch. Plus, with lighter weights you can perform more repetitions, which may enhance cardio burn.

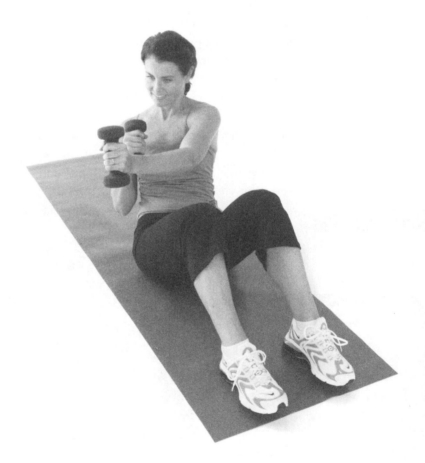

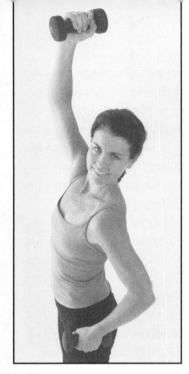

before you begin

Perhaps you've gotten very out of shape or you're returning to fitness after an injury or a weighty pregnancy. Maybe you're feeling "too old" or "too unathletic" to be fit. I'm here to nip all that naysaying in the bud. You can do it. I've seen some amazing transformations over the years and they prove that it's never too late to embark on a fitness program. So think positively. Being fit and trim is possible, no matter what shape you're in now.

Here is a list of guidelines to consider as you begin using *Weights for Weight Loss*:

Get medical clearance from your doctor. You must be sure that your basic health is good before starting your fitness program.

Start conservatively. Read through the pages of this book and ingest all its ideas. Then as you begin the workouts, use the lightest of weights, or no weights at all.

Make an appointment for fitness, just like you make an appointment to get your hair cut. Put it in your daily planner—in ink. For many people,

just finding the time is the major obstacle and could be the reason for their lack of fitness in the first place.

Focus on form and alignment. Study the pictures closely and read the exercise descriptions.

Never hold your breath, and pay attention to your breathing throughout your workouts. If you feel very out of breath and your heart is racing, try to calm your body and mind by stopping the exercise and standing upright in place. You may also want to take a sip of water at this point. Try not to lie or sit down, as this may

cause your heart rate to drop too drastically, which can make you feel dizzy or nauseated.

Avoid eating two hours before exercise. There are two reasons for this. One, you'll have the most energy because no energy will be going toward digestion. And two, you'll be most comfortable. Exercising on a full stomach is very unpleasant.

Invest in a good pair of cross-training sneakers. You want your feet to be stable and cushioned (especially for the jump-rope series). A cross-trainer sneaker will be ideal for walking, biking, running, ten-

18

nis and other cardio activities too.

Recruit a workout buddy to make things more interesting and to keep you on your fitness path. I know that as a personal trainer, I've been a glorified workout buddy for many of my clients. They know what to do and how to do it, but they need someone to help them keep their workout promise. Having the support of a friend, coworker, relative or spouse can make a huge difference, and people are a lot less likely to cancel a workout if they know they'll have to answer to someone else.

Be sure to warm up a little before grabbing those weights. The next section contains specific advice about warming up before you work out.

Warming Up

Because the potential for injury increases when the body is cold, cardiovascular activity is the preliminary tool for a warm-up. The idea of taking five minutes to "warm up" is to raise the core temperature of your body and your muscles. A warm-up should consist of a light aerobic activity that uses the muscles you plan on exercising during your workout. A proper warm-up lubricates the joints, warms the connective tissues and stimulates the nervous and the circulatory systems. According to the American Council on Exercise (ACE), a warm-up helps to prevent injury by improving the elasticity of muscles.

A general warm-up can be any light, continuous movement using the large muscle groups, like marching or jogging in place, or slowly jumping rope. You can hop on a stationary bicycle or treadmill, or go for a walk around the block. Whatever warm-up you choose should produce a small amount of perspiration but shouldn't leave you feeling fatigued. Actually, you should feel invigorated, ready to progress into the workout.

Get Moving with Cardio

With modern life becoming increasingly sedentary, adding cardiovascular exercise into your routine is vital to your overall well-being. For this rea-

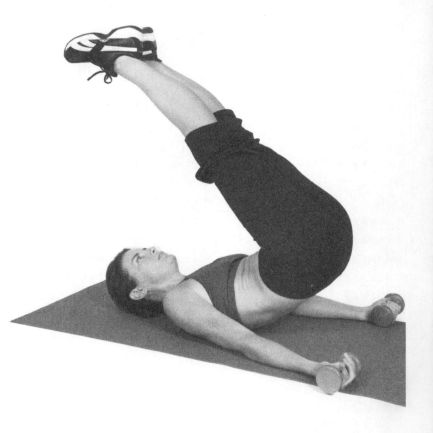

son, even the weight-training workouts in this book have at least a splash of cardio.

Cardiovascular exercise is an activity that raises your heart rate to a level where it feels like you're working. It's a great way to burn a lot of calories in a little time. It gets your blood pumping, so your circulation thrives. It strengthens your heart and increases your lung capacity. It makes you feel good and sleep better. Studies prove that it helps drastically reduce stress. Cardio is an all-natural wonder drug. If you're not taking advantage of it, start right now! Hop on the treadmill or sign up for a dance class. Cardio activity can greatly improve your quality of life, and it can fit into your everyday life in an assortment of ways.

Stuck at the office? Take the stairs. Going shopping? Park your car far away. Hanging out at home? Housework, gardening and home repair are all great cardiovascular activities. I live in an urban environment where I walk to the post office, the Italian deli, the bank, the coffee shop and my studio. I have a dog, too, so I'm always walking. One day I wore my friend's pedometer and tracked my mileage…8,000 paces! (No wonder I sleep so soundly.) This is a great example of how

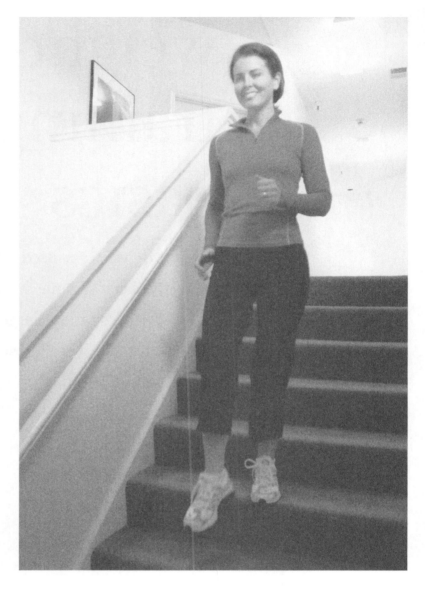

little activities throughout the day can really add up.

The drive-through is just so convenient, I know. So is getting food delivered, or hiring a housekeeper, or letting the valet park the car. Modern life is full of shortcuts that can contribute to obesity and poor

health. Get in the habit of taking the *less easy* option physically. Especially if you aren't able get to the gym. Every energized, slim person I know moves a lot throughout their day. Energy begets energy. Use it and you'll acquire more of it.

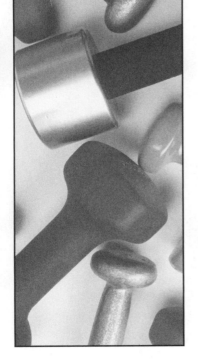

weight-training basics

Maybe you've never used handheld weights, or maybe it's been a while since you have. To make sure everyone's on the same page regarding weight-training protocol, here are several important things to know before you begin pumping iron.

Choosing a Weight

Although Nautilus-type machines are useful for strength training, *Weights for Weight Loss* utilizes free weights so you can work out anywhere—at home, at the gym or while traveling. Free weights are individual, hand-held weights, and they can be purchased in a set of varied sizes or by the pair. They can be steel, rubber-encased or vinyl, and they come in an array of colors.

Selecting the composition and color of your weights comes down to personal preference. You may like the way the rubber-encased weights don't harm a hardwood floor, or the fact that the vinyl ones have a less slippery grip. Personally, I

think the various bright colors are fun and serve a valuable function: I can look down and know which size is which just by the color. Blue is 5 pounds, purple 7 pounds, etc. This is especially handy if you find yourself changing your weights often during your workout.

Choosing appropriate sizes for your weights is crucial; one size does not fit all! I liken size selection to test-driving a car. It comes down to feel and function. I think it's best to have at least three sets of weights on hand. You'll need four sets for the workouts in this book.

The first set, called the *light pair*, is for when you want to go slightly faster and perform more repetitions, or "reps."

With the light pair, you should be able to do 20 reps before you feel fatigue.

With the second set, called the *middle pair*, you should feel fatigue by around rep number 12. (The middle pair is very versatile, and if you're traveling and can only bring along one set of weights, I recommend this pair.)

The third set of weights, or the *heavy pair*, is especially for our Super Sculpt exercises, where you want to exhaust the muscles of the body with fewer repetitions—you definitely should be tired by repetition number 10.

Specifically for Slow-Motion Chisel, we take the *heaviest pair* up one notch—maybe a pound or two heavier than the "heavy pair." The heaviest pair should allow for 5 tough but good reps. Your muscle should want to call it quits by repetition number 8. See the Weight-Selection Chart above for a quick overview.

In general, the weight must be challenging to the muscle but absolutely do-able. You should be able to perform a full range of motion. It's always better to start off with resistance that's too easy than too hard. If you are straining and the weight is too much, the chance of injuring yourself is higher. In this book, I use a 3-pound set, a 5-pound set, a 7-pound set and an 8-pound set. Keep in mind that as you get stronger the weights will seem lighter, and reevaluating your four sets of weights will be important. For example, over time, your "heaviest" pair may become your "heavy" pair.

GET A GRIP!

The way you hold free weights is important. Clenching too tightly wastes energy and may cause the neck, wrist and forearms to burn out unnecessarily. On the flip side, holding on too loosely may increase the risk of dropping the weight or performing the exercise erratically. Find a happy medium. Somewhere in between too tight and too loose is just right.

WEIGHT-SELECTION CHART

WEIGHTS	# OF REPS	PACE	WORKOUT
light pair	many	fast	*Cardio/Sculpt Circuit*
middle pair	medium	slower or faster	*Cardio/Sculpt Circuit* or *Body Blitz*
heavy pair	few	fairly slow	*Body Blitz* or *Super Sculpt*
heaviest pair	very few	very slow	*Slow-Motion Chisel*

Breathing

There are three rules of thumb when it comes to breathing while working out. First and foremost is to *keep breathing*. The worst thing you can do when weight training is to hold your breath. Second, focus on the exhale. A strong exhale will provoke a strong inhale, and the supply of oxygen in the bloodstream will be magical since this helps the muscle rejuvenate on the spot. Third, exhale on exertion. By exertion I mean the most trying part of the movement, when the muscle is fully engaged.

In each of the exercise descriptions, I've written a breathing pattern that coincides with the movement, so be sure to pay attention to those cues, especially during your first run-through.

Core Stabilization

The core muscles (the abdominal, internal and external obliques, the transverse abdominus, and the lower back muscles) need to be slightly engaged in order for you to do each exercise safely. Without stabilization, the spine may be taxed to an undesirable degree and the exercises will feel and look sloppy. Stabilizing the core is a cinch. Pretend you are wearing a corset or a tight-fitting outfit. Pull your navel to your spine, lift the ribcage off the waist and feel the muscles of the core "hug" the spinal column. Every exercise in this book requires core stabilization.

Control

I probably remind people 20 times per day, "No momentum." This is for safety reasons as well as function. Excessive momentum precipitates injuries. Swinging movements alone are hazardous, but combined with extra weight they can lead to disaster in the form of strains, sprains and dislocations. Furthermore, excessive momentum contributes to unbalanced muscular development because only one part of the muscle gets the appropriate resistance. The ends of the exercise—the bottom and the top positions—receive either too little or too much resistance. Avoiding momentum by slowing down the movement leads to safer full-range resistance, so please keep all movements under control.

Mental Focus

Without mental focus, the body can be trained, but it cannot be trained *perfectly*. By perfectly, I mean efficiently, safely and symmetrically. Consequently, mental focus is required for all of the exercises featured in this book. Just like an athlete amidst competition, you need a form of concentration that is consistently in the moment. (You shouldn't be thinking about what's for dinner!) The mind is the real builder of the body—action follows thought. Aspire to stay on the task at hand and the results of these workouts will be more pleas-

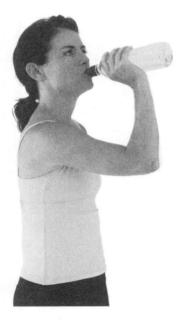

ing. Once you establish mental focus, all of the other aspects in this section (breathing, core stabilization, control) will also fall into place without much effort.

Rest

Don't overtrain! The one big misconception in exercise is the belief that more is more. It's like doubling up on your medication to get better more quickly. If you work out too hard, too long or without proper rest, you'll end up doing more harm to your body than good. There are limits of muscular endurance. Violating those limits causes injury, low energy and an overall feeling of irritation. This applies to the amount of weight you lift, the duration for which you work out, and the frequency with which you work out. Everything has to be *balanced*.

Taking some time out for rest and recovery is fundamental to anyone interested in fitness, and particularly for people involved in weight training. To help you understand why, here's a short description of what happens to muscles during exertion: When muscles contract, their microscopic fibers slide over one another. With sufficient muscular stimulus, such as when you are lifting a weight, these fibers pull apart, causing

TIPS FOR MENTAL FOCUS

- Work out with the TV off.
- Turn off your cellular phone and, if you're at home, turn off the landline ringers.
- Connect to the breath as much as possible. Pay attention to the inhale and the exhale.
- Listening to music may be beneficial in that it can block out distracting noises, but choose CDs not radio. The radio, with its advertisements and interludes of chitchat can disturb your mental focus.
- Organize your space so everything you may need—water bottle, weights, exercise mat, towel—is all together, in one place.
- Keep pets away. This may seem strange to mention, but dogs especially can disturb your lifting flow.
- Count your reps—out loud, in a whisper (as you exhale), or in your head.

trauma at a microscopic level. The body responds to this stress by rebuilding the bridges between the fibers. The body repairs itself to be slightly stronger than it was before, so that next time it will be able to manage the challenge more effectively.

You don't really need to remember this, but you *do* need to remember that the building-up part happens *between*, not *during*, workouts. When your body is at rest, it is actually getting a lot accomplished. How often you should weight-train depends on your overall health and your current lifestyle, and this varies from person to person. Most people can make excellent progress with three to four workouts per week. Just be sure to sleep well, and always take one complete day off every week.

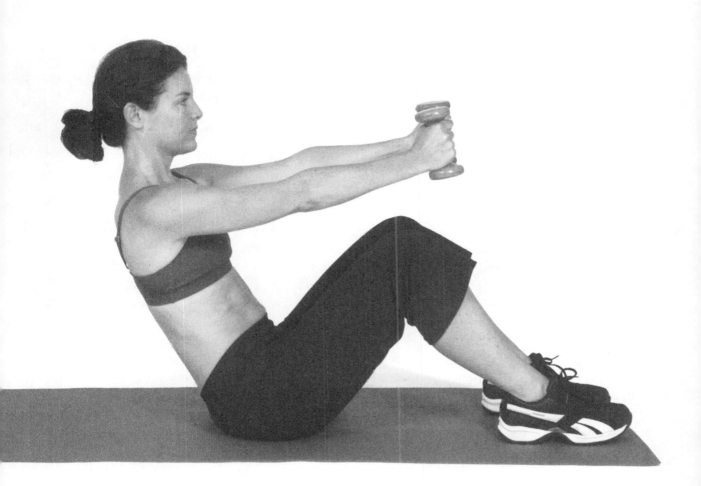

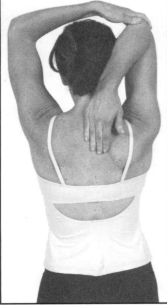

other workout essentials

We've already established that a balanced weight-training workout combined with a balanced diet is the key to losing weight and keeping it off. Your routine should include core work as well as stretching to make it complete.

Core Workout with Weights

Your core muscles are just like all the other muscles in your body, so you should train them the same way you would train, say, your biceps or your chest. At the end of each of the four weight-loss workouts, I recommend three core exercises for a more thorough total-body challenge. However, you can select any of the core exercises from Part 3 and perform them alone as a quick ab-blaster.

Adding weights to abdominal exercises is an exciting way to get more intensity with each repetition, but I assure you that the core exercises in Part 3 are challenging even without the added resistance. So, especially if you're new to this, perform them without weights if need be. Many of these exercises are Pilates-inspired, making them truly about the *entire* core—front, back and sides—and very balanced. A balanced core is a highly functional one.

Stretching

Now you've worked hard. Perhaps you're sweating! Your muscles are warm and elastic. It's time to work on flexibility by stretching. Stretching is such a sweet reward—a time to tend peacefully to the elongation of your muscles. Static stretching, when one muscle group is targeted and gradually stretched, is the sensible thing to do at this point of your workout for two key reasons. One, it helps break up and clear out the lactic acid produced by working muscles, allowing the muscles to recover with less (or no) soreness. Two, stretching is also believed to help prevent injury to tendons, ligaments and muscles by improving muscular elasticity and tone.

In Part 3 I showcase several stretches for the major muscles of the body. As with everything else in this book, be balanced with your stretch series. Hit lower and upper body muscles evenly. Also, hold stretches for at least 30 seconds consistently.

Hamstrings, lower back, quadriceps, chest and shoulders tend to be ideal areas to focus on after weight training because they are the major muscles involved with the movements. Be sure to eliminate excess shoulder and neck tension, too, with simple shoulder rolls and neck circles. These can be done during and after your workout to keep tension at bay.

Static stretching is slow, controlled and safe. Ballistic stretching is jerky, bouncy and can be dangerous, because momentum takes over and control is lost. Make sure your stretches are static, as opposed to ballistic. I find if you slow down and deepen your breathing as you stretch, your chances of stretching statically are greater.

Stretching can be an art form, and there are entire books exclusively devoted to stretching. I recommend obtaining a book about stretching if you are interested in delving deeper into the mechanics.

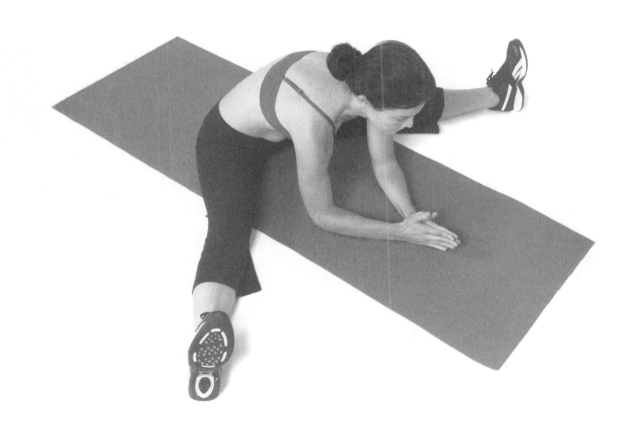

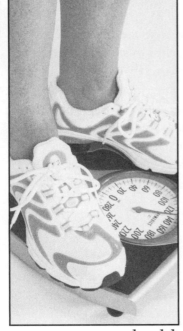

keeping it off

Weight-loss success is not an accident—it's a good habit. Stick with it. I'm talking about hanging in there! It may take a month or so to see subtle results, so be patient. You've started something that I hope you'll continue, even after the numbers on the scale match up with your ideal. It'll start to feel easier and easier to maintain a healthy weight when you are more naturally inclined to do so. As I mentioned earlier, I do think it is worse to lose and regain than never to have lost at all. Take it off and keep it off with persistence!

Dodging the Dreaded Plateau

However, even if you are consistent in keeping your "good habit," you may find you have reached a weight-loss plateau. In relation to losing weight and working out, "plateau" might as well be a four-letter word. But what does the plateau really mean? Is it all in our heads? A plateau, in general, is a stubborn standstill. A *weight-loss plateau* is when the body finds a comfortable weight to maintain. Many people in the midst of dropping, say, 50 pounds, hit a plateau just when those last seven pounds need to come off. When it comes to dieting, this plateau is very real, and it can be extremely frustrating. What really happens is this: by losing weight, you've told your body to just stop burning fuel, to prepare itself for a period of famine. Our bodies are programmed to prevent weight loss for survival. Thus your metabolism is lowered in an attempt to slow the use of your fatty energy reserves.

The way to dodge a weight-loss plateau is very straightforward—you must increase your activity level. This will boost your metabolism, and your body will continue to burn energy at a nice clip. This is why diet and exercise go hand in hand. Dieting without exercise produces insufficient results, especially when it gets down to those last few pounds.

Another common plateau is the *workout* plateau, which is a fitness rut. The human body is very efficient and quickly adapts to any workload. Once the body practices the same activity repeatedly, it grows more proficient at performing that activity. Thus, it requires less energy and therefore less of a caloric burn.

By spending the past 15 years in the gym, I've learned that this plateau is a bit exaggerated. Sure, everything gets easier, but some challenge is still there; your body is just meeting the challenge with less effort. It may not feel as intense, but the workout isn't worthless—you're still benefiting. And the really good news is this: dodging this type of plateau is a cinch, especially with this book, because variety is the solution.

In Part 2 I present four workout plans in *Weight for Weight Loss*, along with three weight-loss programs. It's very unlikely that you'll get into a workout rut if you follow the protocol established in this book. Just increasing the amount of weight of your handheld weights can prevent a plateau.

So yes, weight-loss and workout plateaus do exist, but they don't have to exist *for you*. You now know how to dodge them—just keep moving and seek variety.

Maintenance

Losing weight and *getting* fit are not much different from *maintaining* weight and *staying* fit. You've got to keep up your regimen. It may sound corny, but fitness is not a destination; it's a journey. When you get to the top of the fitness mountain and say, "Oh, I've made it. Now I can stop," you are sabotaging your hard-earned wellness. This very common conclusion is detrimental to the maintenance of your fabulous newfound physique and is simply not true. We mustn't stop. We are always climbing. Exercise is a lifetime commitment.

If for some reason you must undergo a prolonged period of inactivity because of travel, injury or another circumstance, don't fret. Just like getting into shape took time, getting out of shape will not happen overnight! Just be disciplined. If exercise isn't happening because of overtime at work, be extra attentive to diet. Try to eat cleanly. On the flipside, if you decide to splurge on desserts or a big late-night meal, put a workout at the top of your to-do list. Once you've attained the right weight and a fit body, there is definitely more room for some give and take.

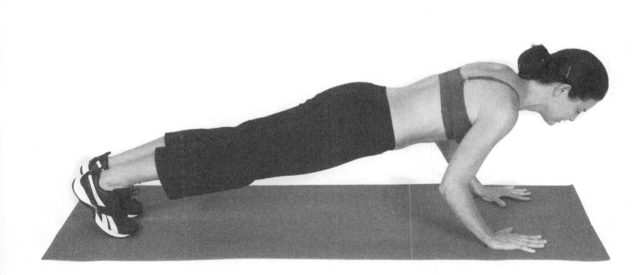

part two:

the

programs

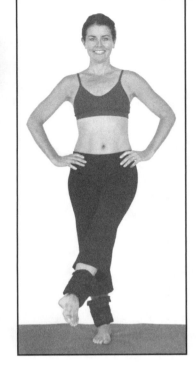

an overview

Part 2 lays out four different workouts and three weight-loss programs, each with a different duration and focus to help you achieve your goal. In addition to challenging your muscles and boosting your metabolism (thus enhancing weight loss), this variety will keep you interested and prevent your body from reaching frustrating plateaus.

The Workouts

When it comes to weight training, many people undertrain their legs and overtrain their upper body or vice versa. An imbalanced workout results in an ill-proportioned body that doesn't function fluidly. In *Weights for Weight Loss*, we are balanced in our training approach, thus making the body look and move better. The four workouts in this section not only meet our overall goal for weight loss, they also promote symmetry by targeting the entire body.

Terminology

Rep is short for "repetition." A rep is the completed range of motion for an exercise. For example, doing one hammer curl would be one rep.

A **set** is the number of reps of a particular exercise that one does before resting or moving on to another exercise. For example, 12 hammer curl reps make up one set.

A **rest interval** is the amount of time taken between sets.

10-Minute Body Blitz

This workout is ideal for when you are time-crunched or in need of an energy jolt. Here, even the busiest person can squeeze in a weight-training workout and accumulate a bit of pep at the same time. You'll efficiently tone the body from head to toe, while simultaneously rev up the active metabolism rate with a burst of cardio.

20-Minute Slow-Motion Chisel

The goal of this workout is to safely exhaust the muscles of the body using a maximum amount of weight at a very slow pace.

30-Minute Super Sculpt

Super Sculpt is the classic weight-training routine that thoroughly tends to every major muscle in the body. The pace is moderate—not too slow yet not too fast—and we aim for a higher amount of weight combined with a lower amount of repetitions.

40-Minute Cardio/Sculpt Circuit

This workout is great for when you wish to kill two birds with one stone. Cardio/Sculpt Circuit combines the best of both worlds (cardiovascular and strength training) by including jump rope. Here the exercises are performed at a fast pace and in a "loop." with no intended rest in between sets in order to keep our fat-burning heart rate elevated.

The Weight-Loss Programs

When it comes to weight loss, one size does not fit all. *Weights for Weight Loss* acknowledges this fact by including three weight-loss programs (see pages 54–55) that incorporate all of the workouts in this book. Choose the one that best meets your needs and goals.

7-Day Weight-Loss Program

Maybe you're preparing for a special event—a wedding, an important presentation, a photo shoot—and you need to look extra sleek. This seven-day

program serves as a countdown to a big day. It includes a form of cardio exercise everyday in order to keep your energy on high all day, everyday. In this program, there's no time for a day off, but I assume Day Eight will be a day of rest from any formal workout.

14-Day Weight-Loss Program

Two weeks is plenty of time to start developing a bit more muscle mass, so the weight loss that occurs during this 14-day period will help pave the way for easier weight management down the road. And don't be fooled—the three days of rest in this program are strategically placed. Your body will actually get a lot accomplished on those days, rejuvenating itself and getting set for the following three days of challenge. Remember, weight loss is our goal, so burning more calories than we consume is the most important factor. Diet plays a

huge role and rest is crucial, especially when working muscles. Without proper rest, you won't be able to conjure up your best effort.

30-Day Weight-Loss Program

This program is all about steady weight loss. You really don't want to lose more than two pounds per week. Any more than that two pounds ends up being water and/or muscle mass loss, which will slow your basal metabolic rate in the long run—the exact opposite of your goal. The 30-day program requires more dedication and planning than the other two programs because I'm asking for more of your time, so be sure to embark on the program when you know you can give it your all, with few distractions. Also, be sure to pull out a calendar and make daily appointments for your workouts.

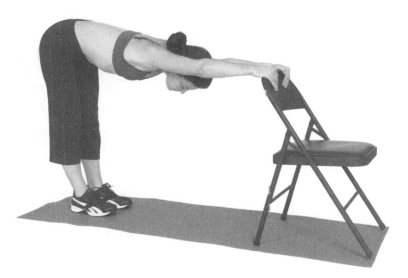

10-minute body blitz

The Body Blitz hits all the major muscles just once with one set of repetition to fatigue. This routine is performed at a robust pace with no official rest in between exercises; sometimes, two exercises are performed simultaneously. Once you complete each of the exercises in the order given, move on to the recommended abdominal exercises, then remember to stretch (see pages 98–105).

WEIGHTS: Use your "middle pair."

PACE & REST: Fairly speedy, like a brisk walk. Move from one exercise to the next quickly, without rest.

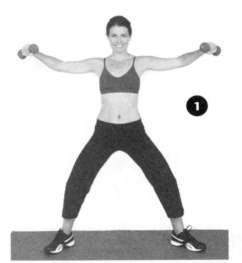

Lateral Raise
(page 64)
1 set of 15 reps

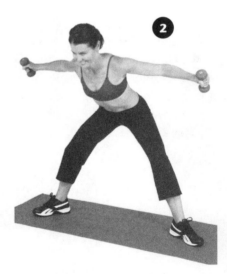

Rear Shoulder Flye
(page 68)
1 set of 15 reps

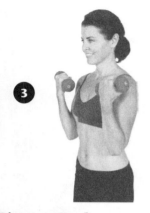

3

Biceps Curl
(page 58)
1 set of 15 reps

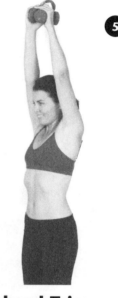

5

Overhead Triceps Press
(page 61)
1 set of 15 reps

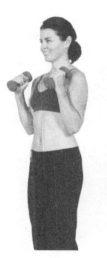

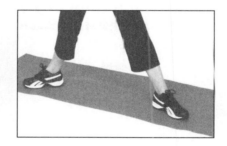

4

Hammer Curl in Wide Plie
(pages 59 & 78)
1 set of 15 reps

10-minute body blitz (continued)

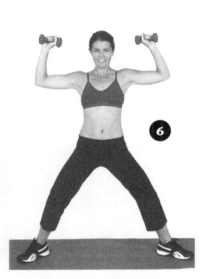

6

Lat Pull Down
(page 69)
1 set of 15 reps

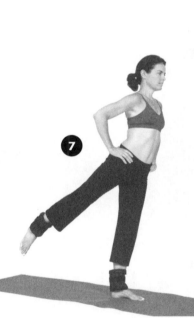

7

**Standing Leg
Extension Back**
(page 80)
1 set of 15 reps

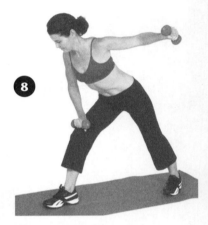

8

**Reverse Flye
Long Arm**
(page 71)
1 set of 15 reps

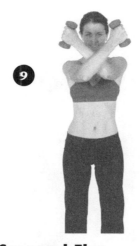

9

Scooped Flye
(page 73)
1 set of 15 reps

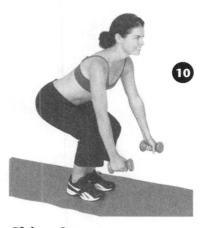

10

Skier Squat
(page 76)
1 set of 15 reps

10-minute body blitz (continued)

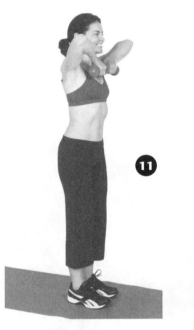

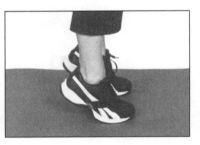

**Upright Row
with Calf Raise
Parallel**

(pages 65 & 84)

1 set of 15 reps

abdominals 1

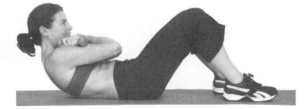

Center Crunch
(page 86)
10 reps

abdominals 2

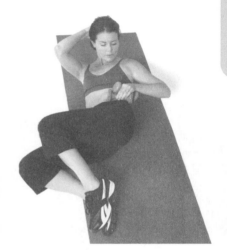

Side Crunch
(page 87)
10 reps each side

abdominals 3

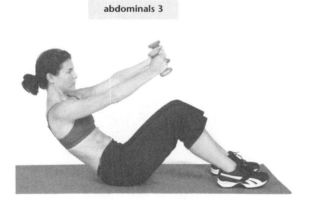

The Teaser
(page 89)
10 reps

20-minute slow-motion chisel

The heaviest weights are used in Slow-Motion Chisel, making way for major resistance. Because of the high levels of resistance, there is no need for a lot of repetition—achieving a double-digit range will be arduous and is totally unexpected in *one* set, but we do attain double digits in *two* sets, thanks to a relatively long rest interval in between. Once you complete all sets of each exercise in the order given, move on to the recommended abdominal exercises, then remember to stretch (see pages 98–105).

WEIGHTS: Use the "heaviest pair."

PACE & REST: Slow-to-moderate pace; the rest interval should be at least 30 seconds, but no more than 45 seconds.

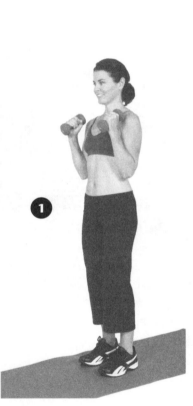

1

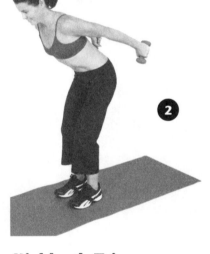

2

3

Kickback Triceps Press
(page 62)

2 sets of 7 reps, with 30–45 seconds rest in between

Hammer Curl
(page 59)

2 sets of 7 reps, with 30–45 seconds rest in between

Upright Row
(page 65)

2 sets of 7 reps, with 30–45 seconds rest in between

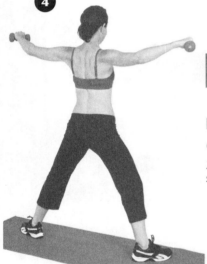

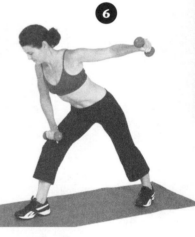

Lat Pull Side

(page 70)

2 sets of 7 reps, with 30–45 seconds rest in between

Upright Raise from Rear

(page 67)

2 sets of 7 reps, with 30–45 seconds rest in between

Reverse Flye Long Arm

(page 71)

2 sets of 7 reps, with 30–45 seconds rest in between

20-minute slow-motion chisel (continued)

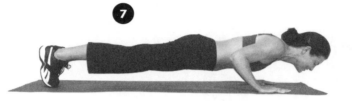

7

Push-Up

(page 74)

2 sets of 7 reps, with 30–45
seconds rest in between

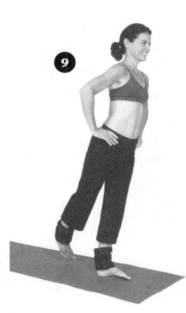

9

Standing Leg Circle

(page 81)

2 sets of 7 reps, with 30–45
seconds rest in between

8

Diagonal Lunge

(page 75)

2 sets of 7 reps, with 30–45
seconds rest in between

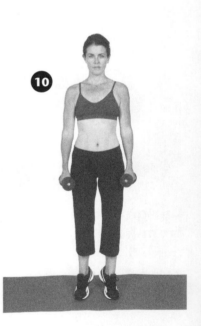

10

Calf Raise Turn-Out

(page 85)

2 sets of 7 reps, with 30–45
seconds rest in between

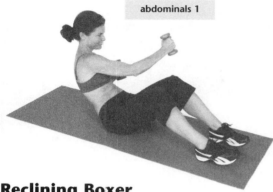

abdominals 1

Reclining Boxer
(page 91)
20 reps total

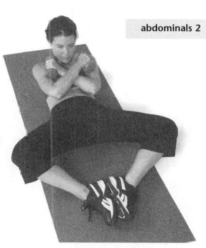

abdominals 2

Diamond Crunch
(page 90)
15 reps

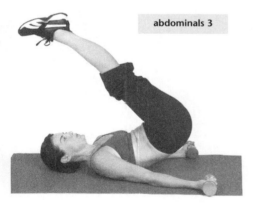

abdominals 3

Hip Lift
(page 88)
10 reps

30-minute super sculpt

"Three" is the magic number as we take three sets of three exercises at a time, aiming for reps of 10, 8 and 6, in that order. Every part of this formula, from the pace to the sequencing, allows for maximum strength challenge. Once you complete all sets of each exercise in the order given, move on to the recommended abdominal exercises, then remember to stretch (see pages 98–105).

> **WEIGHTS:** Use the "heaviest pair."
>
> **PACE & REST:** The pace should be medium and steady, like a jog as opposed to a walk or a run. Rest for approximately 10 seconds between each set.

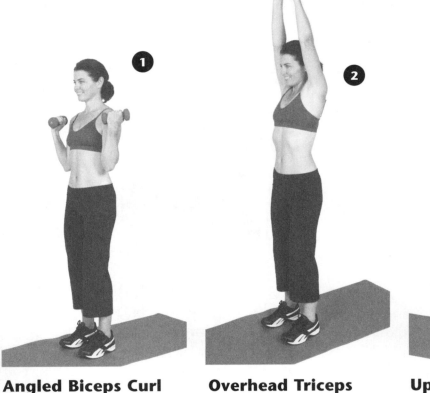

Angled Biceps Curl
(page 60)
set 1: 10 reps
set 2: 8 reps
set 3: 6 reps

Overhead Triceps Press
(page 61)
set 1: 10 reps
set 2: 8 reps
set 3: 6 reps

Upright Row
(page 65)
set 1: 10 reps
set 2: 8 reps
set 3: 6 reps

SEQUENCE FOR EXERCISES 1–3: *Do set 1 for exercises 1–3, then rest for 10 seconds. Do set 2 for exercises 1–3, then rest for 10 seconds. Do set 3 for exercises 1–3, then rest for 10 seconds. Now move on to exercises 4–6.*

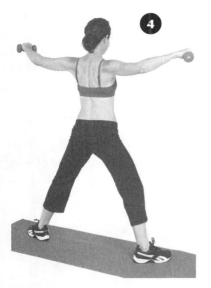

Upright Raise
from Rear

(page 67)

set 1: 10 reps

set 2: 8 reps

set 3: 6 reps

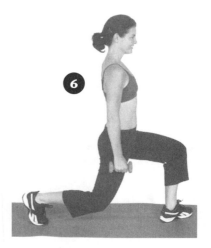

Diagonal Lunge

(page 75)

set 1: 10 reps

set 2: 8 reps

set 3: 6 reps

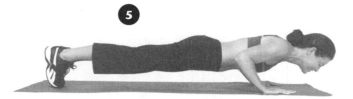

Push-Up

(page 74)

set 1: 10 reps

set 2: 8 reps

set 3: 6 reps

SEQUENCE FOR EXERCISES 4–6: *Do set 1 for exercises 4–6, then rest for 10 seconds. Do set 2 for exercises 4–6, then rest for 10 seconds. Do set 3 for exercises 4–6, then rest for 10 seconds. Now move on to exercises 7–9.*

30-minute super sculpt

30-minute super sculpt (continued)

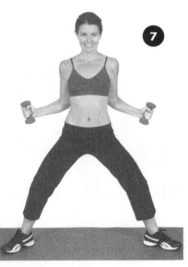

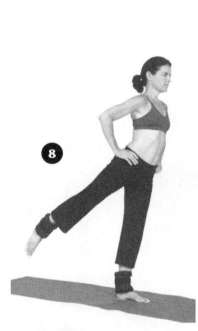

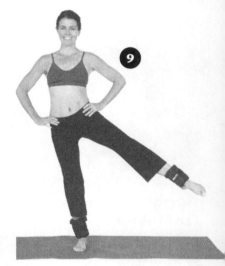

Lat Pull Side

(page 70)

set 1: 10 reps
set 2: 8 reps
set 3: 6 reps

Standing Leg Extension Back

(page 80)

set 1: 10 reps
set 2: 8 reps
set 3: 6 reps

Standing Side Leg Lift

(page 82)

set 1: 10 reps
set 2: 8 reps
set 3: 6 reps

SEQUENCE FOR EXERCISES 7–9: *Do set 1 for exercises 7–9, then rest for 10 seconds. Do set 2 for exercises 7–9, then rest for 10 seconds. Do set 3 for exercises 7–9, then rest for 10 seconds. Now move on to exercises 10–12.*

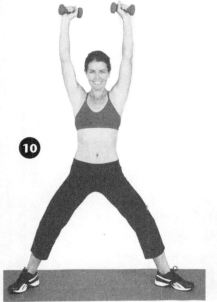

Shoulder Press

(page 66)

set 1: 10 reps
set 2: 8 reps
set 3: 6 reps

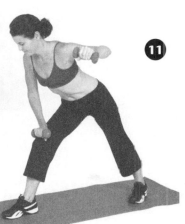

Reverse Flye
Short Arm

(page 72)

set 1: 10 reps
set 2: 8 reps
set 3: 6 reps

The Scissor

(page 83)

set 1: 10 reps
set 2: 8 reps
set 3: 6 reps

30-minute super sculpt

SEQUENCE FOR EXERCISES 10–12: *Do set 1 for exercises 10–12, then rest for 10 seconds. Do set 2 for exercises 10–12, then rest for 10 seconds. Do set 3 for exercises 10–12, then rest for 10 seconds. Now move on to the abdominal exercises.*

30-minute super sculpt (continued)

abdominals 1

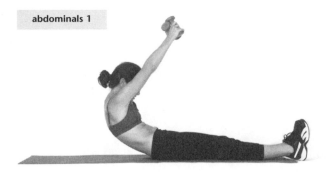

Roll-Up
(page 95)
10 reps

abdominals 2

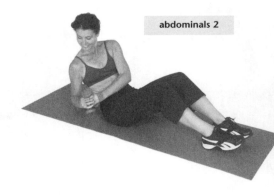

Seated Rowing
(page 94)
20 reps total

abdominals 3

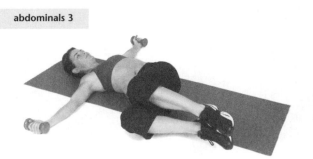

Alternating Knee Drop
(page 92)
20 reps total

40-minute cardio/sculpt circuit

The exercises in this workout are performed at a fast pace (as many reps as you can in 30 seconds) and in a "loop," where we start from the beginning and cycle through the sequence three times. This keeps the heart rate in a good fat-burning zone. We incorporate the jump rope for nine 1-minute intervals (you can increase the interval to 2 minutes each if you have more time). It's nice to have an obvious clock on the wall, a stop watch or a watch with a second hand so you can be more accurate with your intervals. Once you complete all three circuits of each exercise in the order given, move on to the recommended abdominal exercises, then remember to stretch (see pages 98–105).

> **WEIGHTS:** Use either the "light" or "middle" pair.
> **PACE & REST:** Very fast pace. Do as many repetitions as possible within the 30-second interval, with no intended rest between sets.

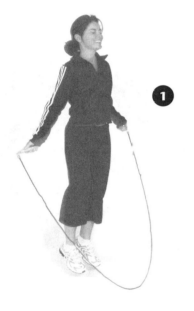

Jump rope

Duration: 1 minute (if you have more time, try to increase the interval to 2 minutes)

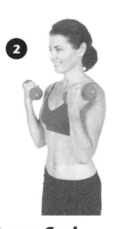

Biceps Curl

(page 58)

Reps: As many as you can in 30 seconds

Shoulder Press

(page 66)

Reps: As many as you can in 30 seconds

40-minute cardio/sculpt circuit

40-minute cardio/sculpt circuit *(continued)*

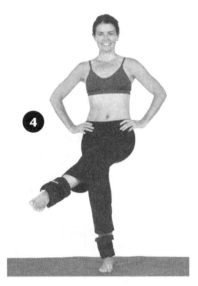

④

The Scissor
(page 83)

Reps: As many as you can in 30 seconds

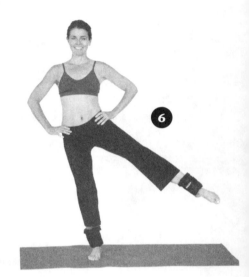

⑥

Standing Side Leg Lift
(page 82)

Reps: As many as you can in 30 seconds

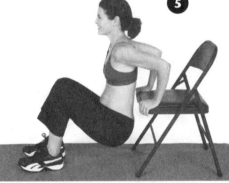

⑤

Triceps Dip
(page 63)

Reps: As many as you can in 30 seconds

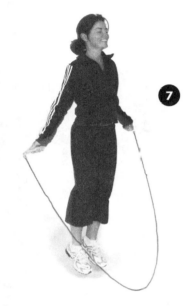

Jump rope

Duration: 1 minute (if you have more time, try to increase the interval to 2 minutes)

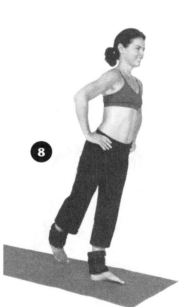

Standing Leg Circle

(page 81)

Reps: As many as you can in 30 seconds

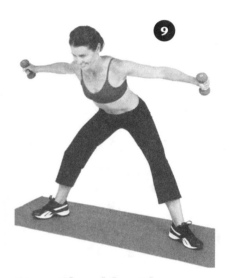

Rear Shoulder Flye

(page 68)

Reps: As many as you can in 30 seconds

40-minute cardio/sculpt circuit

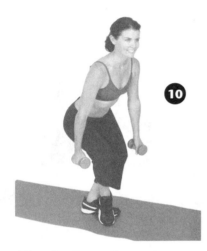

Single-Leg Squat

(page 77)

Reps: As many as you can in 30 seconds

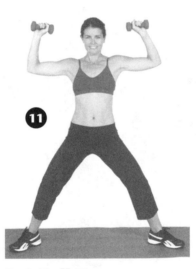

Lat Pull Down

(page 69)

Reps: As many as you can in 30 seconds

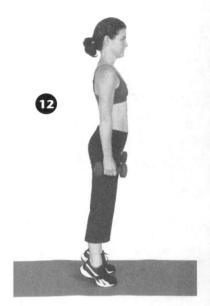

Calf Raise Parallel

(page 84)

Reps: As many as you can in 30 seconds

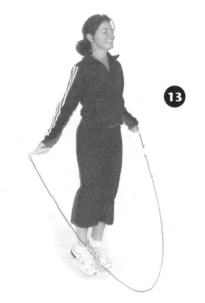

Jump rope

Duration: 1 minute (if you have more time, try to increase the interval to 2 minutes)

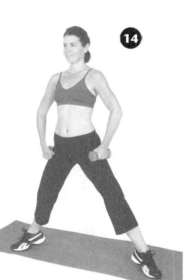

Tip-Toe Plie

(page 79)

Reps: As many as you can in 30 seconds

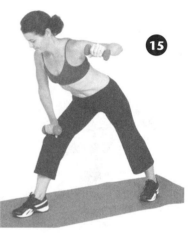

Reverse Flye Short Arm

(page 72)

Reps: As many as you can in 30 seconds

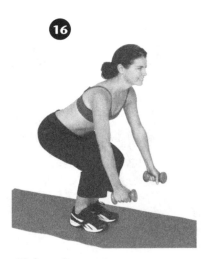

16

Skier Squat

(page 76)

Reps: As many as you can in 30 seconds

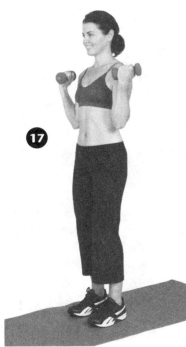

17

Angled Biceps Curl

(page 60)

Reps: As many as you can in 30 seconds

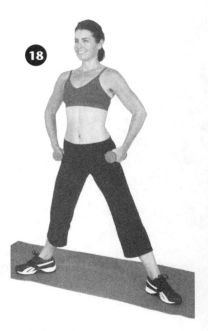

18

Wide Plie

(page 78)

Reps: As many as you can in 30 seconds

Now go back to exercise 1 and cycle through this sequence again until you've done the circuit a total of 3 times.

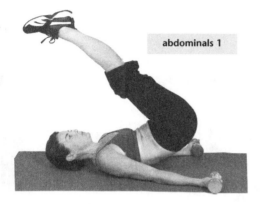

abdominals 1

Hip Lift
(page 88)

10 reps

abdominals 2

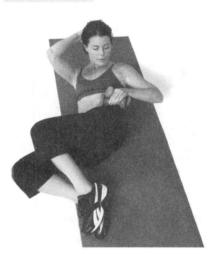

Side Crunch
(page 87)

10 reps each side

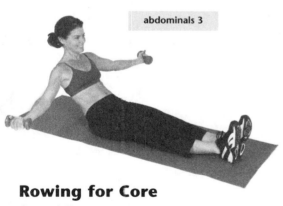

abdominals 3

Rowing for Core
(page 96)

10 reps

the weight-loss programs

7-day weight-loss program

1	2	3	4	5	6	7
Cardio/Sculpt Circuit	Slow-Motion Chisel *extra cardio*	Super Sculpt *extra cardio*	Body Blitz *extra cardio*	Cardio/Sculpt Circuit	Super Sculpt *extra cardio*	Body Blitz *extra cardio*

14-day weight-loss program

1	2	3	4	5	6	7
Super Sculpt *extra cardio*	Cardio/Sculpt Circuit	Body Blitz	**rest & relax!**	Slow-Motion Chisel *extra cardio*	Cardio/Sculpt Circuit	Body Blitz

8	9	10	11	12	13	14
rest & relax!	Super Sculpt *extra cardio*	Cardio/Sculpt Circuit	Body Blitz *extra cardio*	**rest & relax!**	Slow-Motion Chisel *extra cardio*	Cardio/Sculpt Circuit

30-day weight-loss program

(30) 1	(40) 2	(20) 3	(10) 4	5	(30) 6	(10) 7
Super Sculpt *extra cardio*	Cardio/Sculpt Circuit	Slow-Motion Chisel *extra cardio*	Body Blitz *extra cardio*	**rest & relax!**	Super Sculpt	Body Blitz

(30) 8	(40) 9	(20) 10	(10) 11	12	(20) 13	(10) 14
Super Sculpt *extra cardio*	Cardio/Sculpt Circuit	Slow-Motion Chisel *extra cardio*	Body Blitz *extra cardio*	**rest & relax!**	Slow-Motion Chisel	Body Blitz

(30) 15	(40) 16	(20) 17	(10) 18	19	(20) 20	(10) 21
Super Sculpt *extra cardio*	Cardio/Sculpt Circuit	Slow-Motion Chisel *extra cardio*	Body Blitz *extra cardio*	**rest & relax!**	Slow-Motion Chisel	Body Blitz

(30) 22	(40) 23	(20) 24	(10) 25	26	(20) 27	(10) 28
Super Sculpt *extra cardio*	Cardio/Sculpt Circuit	Slow-Motion Chisel *extra cardio*	Body Blitz *extra cardio*	**rest & relax!**	Slow-Motion Chisel	Body Blitz

(30) 29	(40) 30
Super Sculpt *extra cardio*	Cardio/Sculpt Circuit

part three:
the exercises

biceps curl

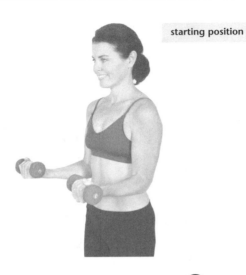

starting position

STARTING POSITION: Stand with your legs hip-width apart and knees slightly bent. Hold one weight in each hand, palms facing up, and bring your elbows in toward your waist. Make a 90-degree angle with your arms, keeping your shoulders down. Engage your abdominals to stabilize the movement. **INHALE** to begin.

1 Moving your arms purely at your elbows and keeping everything else motionless, **EXHALE** and bring the weights toward your shoulders. Be sure to keep the movement under your control and not swing the weights.

2 **INHALE** and return to the starting position.

MODIFICATION

Instead of working both arms simultaneously, alternate one arm at a time.

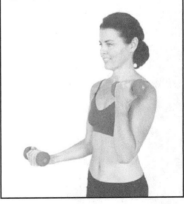

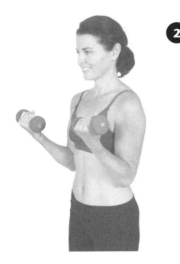

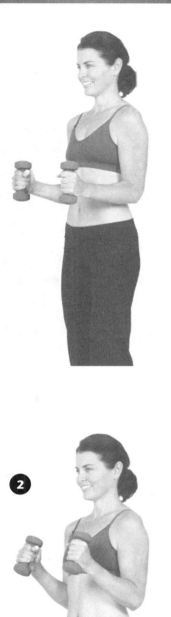

starting position

STARTING POSITION: Stand with your legs hip-width apart and knees slightly bent. Hold one weight in each hand, thumbside up, and bring your elbows in toward your waist. Keep your shoulders down and your core engaged throughout the movement. **INHALE** to begin.

1 **EXHALE** and bend at the elbows, bringing your hands up to shoulder height. Keep everything else motionless.

2 **INHALE** and return to the starting position.

MODIFICATION

Instead of working both arms simultaneously, alternate one arm at a time.

angled biceps curl

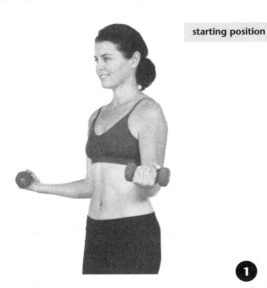

starting position

STARTING POSITION: Stand with your legs hip-width apart and knees slightly bent. Hold one weight in each hand, palms facing up, and bring your elbows in toward the sides of your waist. Angle your forearms to the side, as if you are presenting two serving trays. Keep your shoulders down and your core engaged. **INHALE** to begin.

1 **EXHALE** and bend at the elbows, bringing your hands up to shoulder height.

2 **INHALE** and return to the starting position.

MODIFICATION

Instead of working both arms simultaneously, alternate one arm at a time.

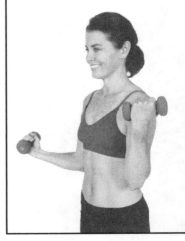

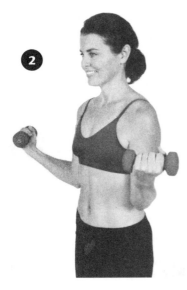

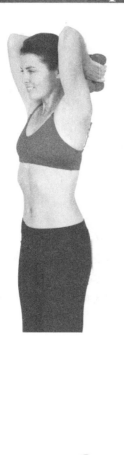

starting position

STARTING POSITION: Stand with your legs hip-width apart and knees slightly bent. Take two weights and combine them so that you're holding them with both hands (or hold one heavier weight with both hands). Raise your arms overhead so that your elbows are by your ears and pointing forward. Keep both elbows bent—this may or may not cause a subtle stretching feeling in your triceps—and lower the weights behind your head. Engage your abdominals. **INHALE** to begin.

1 EXHALE and straighten your elbows, lifting the weight toward the ceiling. Imagine hammering a nail into the ceiling in slow motion. The energy is "up" and the range of motion is big.

2 INHALE and return to the starting position.

kickback triceps press

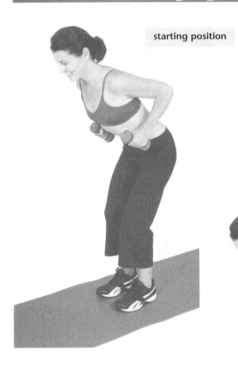

starting position

STARTING POSITION: Stand with your legs hip-width apart and knees slightly bent. Lean your upper body forward and engage your core muscles to keep your back flat throughout the exercise. Now, keeping your arms by your sides, raise both elbows toward the ceiling. **INHALE** to begin.

1 EXHALE and straighten your elbows behind your back, squeezing your triceps as hard as you can. Keep everything else completely still.

2 INHALE and return with control to the starting position.

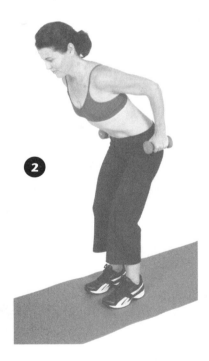

MODIFICATION

Instead of working both arms simultaneously, work one arm at a time, using your knee or a chair for support.

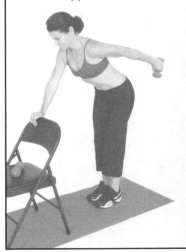

starting position

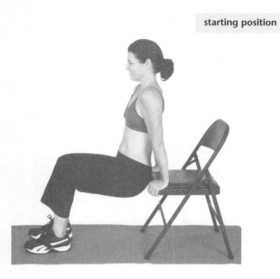

STARTING POSITION: Stand facing away from a stable chair or a bench. Place your hands on the edge of the chair or bench, with your fingers curling over the front of the seat. Bend your knees and plant your feet, forming an "L" with your thighs and torso. Keep your hips and lower back as close to the chair's edge as comfortably possible.

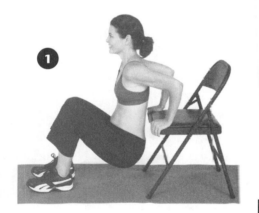

1 INHALE and bend both elbows, dipping your entire body down 3 to 6 inches, never allowing your shoulders to fall below your elbows. Keep your shoulders away from your ears and keep your back close to the chair.

2 EXHALE and push your body back to the starting position.

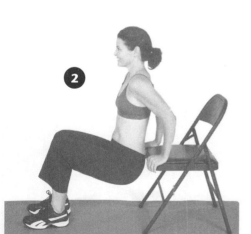

MODIFICATION
Make the movement smaller, dipping down only 1 or 2 inches.

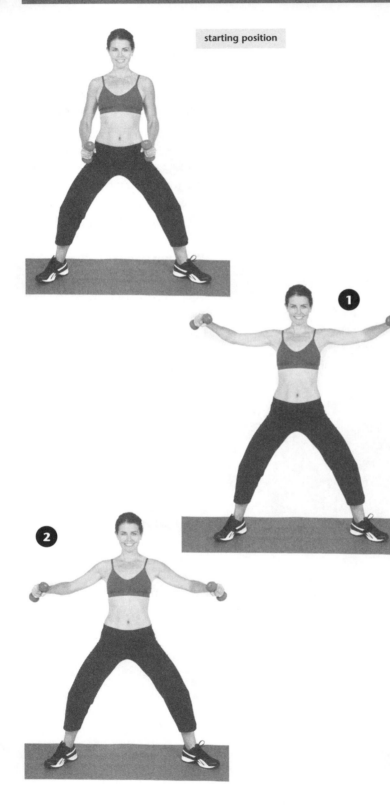

starting position

STARTING POSITION: Stand in a sturdy wide stance—approximately two feet wider than hip-width—and bend your knees slightly. With your arms by your sides, hold one weight firmly in each hand, palms facing your body. Engage your core muscles and drop your shoulders.

1 Keeping a microbend in your elbows, **INHALE** and raise both arms evenly up toward shoulder level. Be sure to keep the wrists firm and the abdominal muscles engaged.

2 **EXHALE** and lower your arms, with control, back to the starting position.

MODIFICATION

Bending your elbows reduces the amount of resistance. So if you feel like the challenge is too great, bend your elbows more.

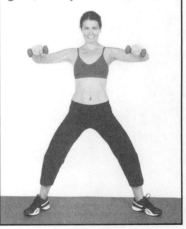

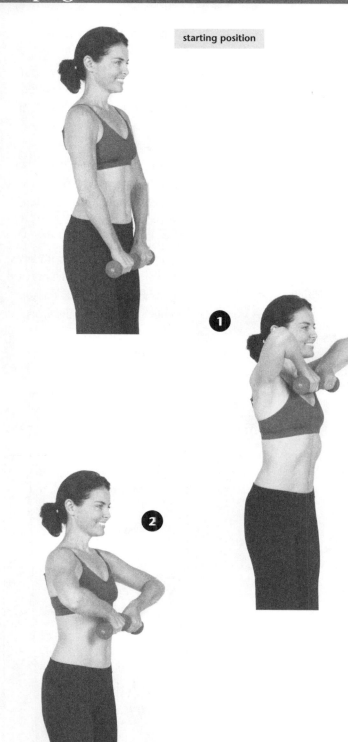

starting position

STARTING POSITION: Stand with your legs hip-width apart and knees slightly bent. Hold one weight in each hand, palms facing the fronts of your thighs. Keep your shoulders down, your core muscles engaged, and your back straight throughout the movement.

1 INHALE and, with your elbows leading the way, raise both weights up to chest level. (Your elbows should always be higher than the weights.) Allow your elbows to jut out to the side and feel your chest lift to a full inhale at the top.

2 EXHALE and lower to the starting position.

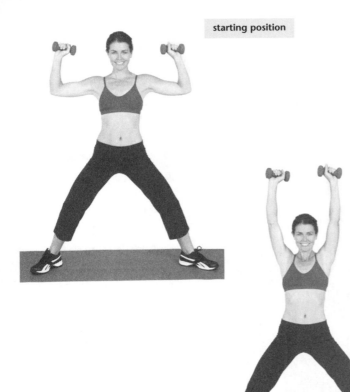

starting position

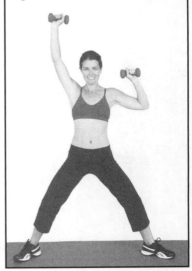

STARTING POSITION: Stand in a sturdy wide stance—approximately two feet wider than hip-width—and bend your knees slightly. Holding a weight in each hand, raise your hands above your shoulders with elbows pointing away from your body. Engage your core muscles and keep your shoulders down. **INHALE** to begin.

1 **EXHALE** and press both arms overhead until the elbows are just about straight. Feel the tops of your shoulders do the work.

2 **INHALE** and return to the starting position.

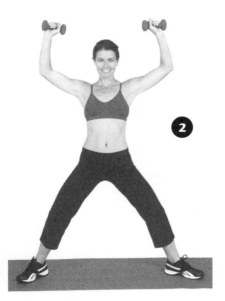

MODIFICATION

Alternate arms, pressing up right, then left.

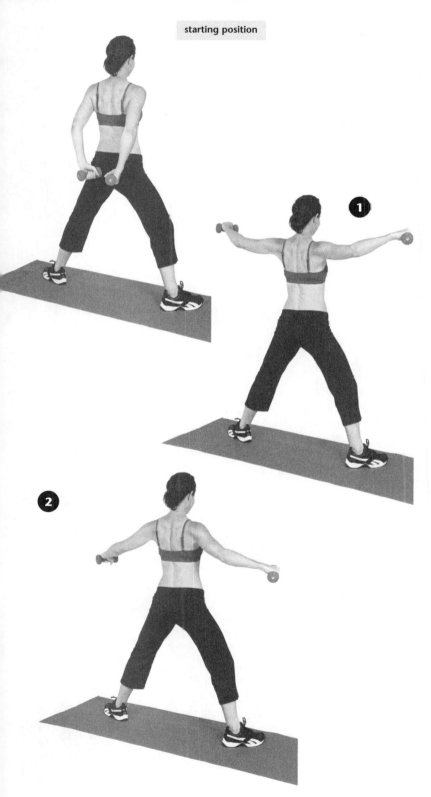

starting position

This exercise is much like Lateral Raise, except the angle of the lift originates at the rear of the body here, rather than the side.

STARTING POSITION: Stand in a sturdy wide stance—approximately two feet wider than hip-width—and bend your knees slightly. With your arms behind you, hold one weight firmly in each hand. Engage your core muscles and drop your shoulders.

1 Keeping a microbend in your elbows, **INHALE** and lift both arms evenly up toward shoulder level. Be sure to keep the wrists firm and the abdominal muscles engaged.

2 **EXHALE** and return, with control, to the starting position.

rear shoulder flye

starting position

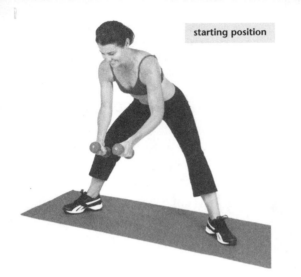

STARTING POSITION: Stand in a sturdy wide stance—approximately three feet apart—and bend your knees slightly. Tilt your upper body forward, keeping your back flat. With your elbows bent, hold your arms out in front of you like bat wings. **INHALE** to begin.

1 **EXHALE** and squeeze your shoulder blades together, as if holding a penny between them.

2 **INHALE** and return to the starting position.

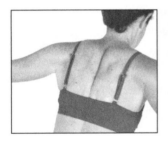

starting position

STARTING POSITION: Stand in a sturdy wide stance—approximately three feet apart—and bend your knees slightly. Stand tall, "stacking" your shoulders over your hips. With one weight in each hand, bring your arms up overhead in a "V." **INHALE** to begin.

1 **EXHALE** and pull the weights down, with control. The movement takes place slightly behind your head.

2 **INHALE** and return to the starting position.

lat pull side

STARTING POSITION: Stand in a sturdy wide stance—approximately three feet apart—and bend your knees slightly. Stand tall, "stacking" your shoulders over your hips. With one weight in each hand, bring your arms up and out to sides, parallel to the floor. **INHALE** to begin.

1 **EXHALE** and pull your elbows in toward your waist. The movement takes place slightly behind your head.

2 **INHALE** and return to the starting position.

starting position

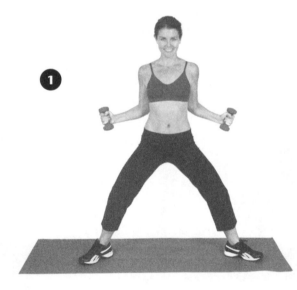

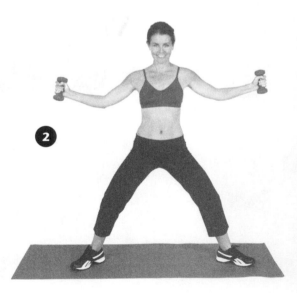

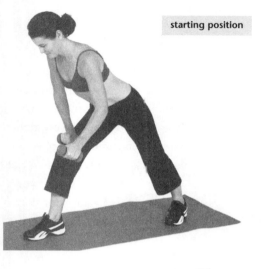

starting position

We'll do one arm at a time to insure the best quality rep possible.

STARTING POSITION: Lunge forward with your right leg, keeping your right knee bent. Lean forward and rest your right hand on your thigh, keeping your back straight. Hold a weight in your left hand in front of your body, keeping your elbow slightly bent. **INHALE** to begin.

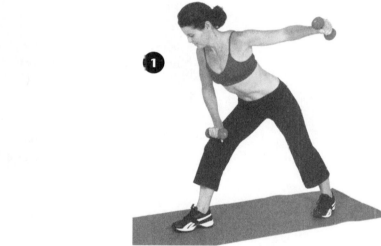

1 Keeping your arm fairly straight and trying to move the arm only at the shoulder, **EXHALE** and press the weight up toward the ceiling. The rest of your body should remain as still as possible.

2 **INHALE** and slowly return to the starting position. Repeat on the other side.

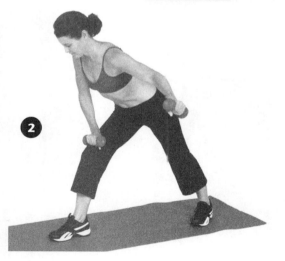

MODIFICATION

If this proves too challenging, perform the Reverse Flye Short Arm (page 72) instead.

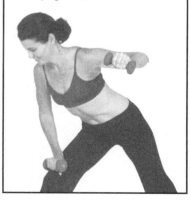

reverse flye short arm

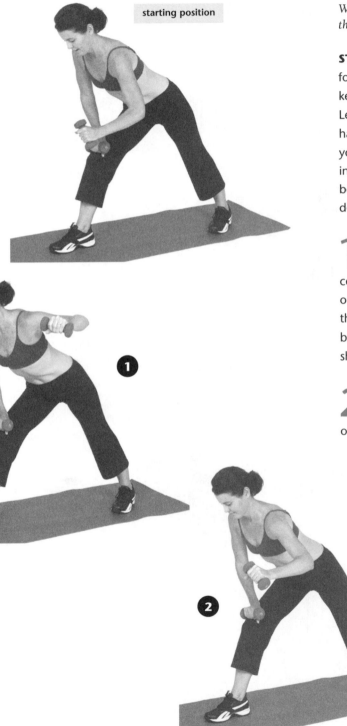

starting position

We'll do one arm at a time to insure the best quality rep possible.

STARTING POSITION: Lunge forward with your right leg, keeping your right knee bent. Lean forward and rest your right hand on your thigh, keeping your back straight. Hold a weight in your left hand in front of your body and bend your elbow 90 degrees. **INHALE** to begin.

1 EXHALE and press your L-shaped arm up toward the ceiling, trying to move the arm only at the shoulder, squeezing the area between your shoulder blades. The rest of your body should remain as still as possible.

2 INHALE and slowly return to the starting position. Repeat on the other side.

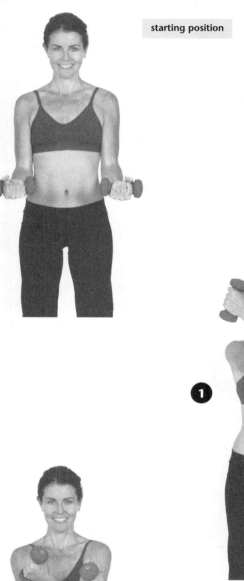

starting position

STARTING POSITION: Plant your feet about hip-width apart and slightly bend both knees. Holding one weight in each hand, bend your elbows 90 degrees and keep your palms up, as if presenting a serving tray. **INHALE** to begin.

1 **EXHALE** and, hinging purely at the shoulder (the elbow stays in a 90-degree bend), push both arms up toward their opposite shoulder, criss-crossing at the forearms. Pretend you're Wonder Woman blocking bullets with your silver bracelets.

2 **INHALE** and return to the starting position. Alternate arms so that your right is over your left, then your left arm is over your right.

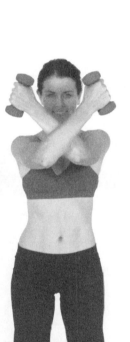

starting position

STARTING POSITION: Bring yourself down to the floor in plank position. Your palms should be positioned directly beneath your shoulders and you should be on the balls of your feet. Press your abdominal muscle up toward your spine to keep your spine straight and your head in a diagonal line with your heels.

1 **INHALE** and bend both of your elbows approximately 90 degrees. Try to keep your elbows in alongside your torso.

2 **EXHALE** and push up to the starting position.

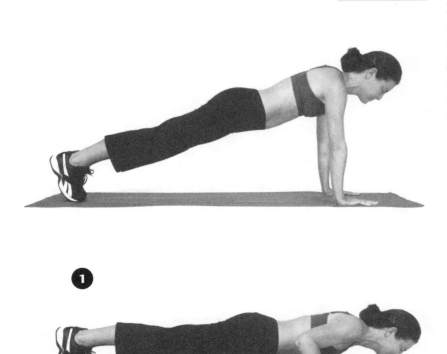

1

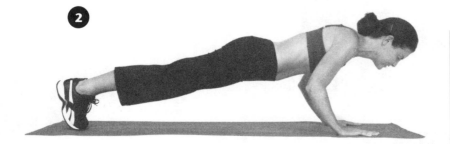

2

MODIFICATION

To lessen the intensity, bend your knees and perform the push-up on your hands and knees instead of the hands and feet.

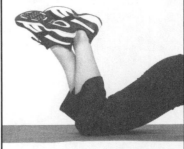

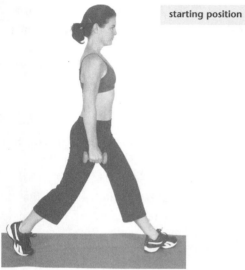

starting position

Here we use the weights as a balance tool and as subtle resistance.

STARTING POSITION: With the left leg, step forward into a slight turn-out, angling your toes slightly away from parallel. Pick up the heel of your back leg (which we call releve in dancer-speak). Keep your shoulders "stacked" over your hips, with the chest lifted and proud. Your arms hang comfortably at your sides with a weight in each hand. **INHALE** to begin.

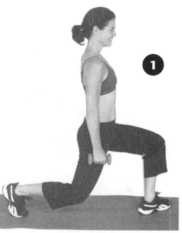

1 **EXHALE** and bend both knees, especially focusing on the dipping of the back knee, as if doing a formal curtsey. Do not compromise your upper body's form (your shoulders must stay over your hips). Imagine that there is a pool of water directly underneath the back knee and you want to test its temperature with your knee cap.

2 **INHALE** and straighten the rear leg back up to the starting position. Switch legs and repeat on the other side.

MODIFICATION

A big challenge with this exercise is balance, so if you'd like extra support, omit the weights and hold onto a wall or the back of a chair.

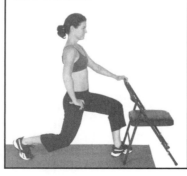

skier squat

target: quadriceps/hamstrings/glutes

STARTING POSITION: Holding one weight in each hand, plant your feet in parallel, close together. Pull your navel toward your spine to engage your core.

1 **INHALE** and bend both knees deeply, keeping the heels of your feet firmly on the floor.

2 **EXHALE** and return to the starting position. Be sure not to round your back.

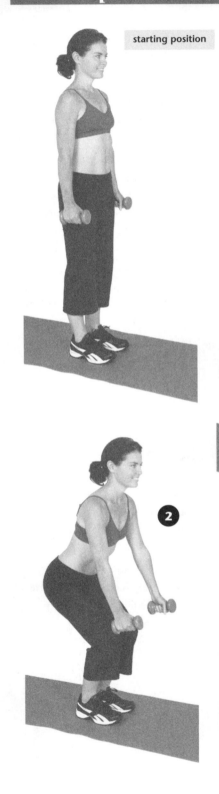

starting position

1

2

MODIFICATION

You can also perform this exercise without weights.

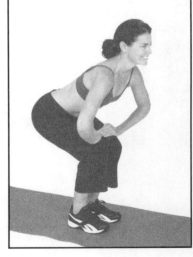

single-leg squat

target: hamstrings/quads/glutes

starting position

STARTING POSITION: Holding one weight in each hand, plant your feet in a turned-out stance with your heels touching. Pick up your right foot and place the heel on top of your left instep.

1 **INHALE** and bend both knees (they should track exactly over the toes), keeping your back completely straight. You should feel as though you're hinging at the hip, not the waist.

2 Using your legs and glutes, **EXHALE** and push yourself back to the starting position. Switch sides.

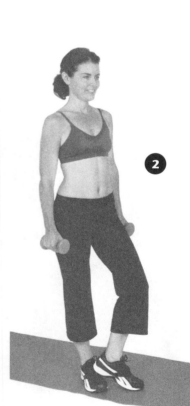

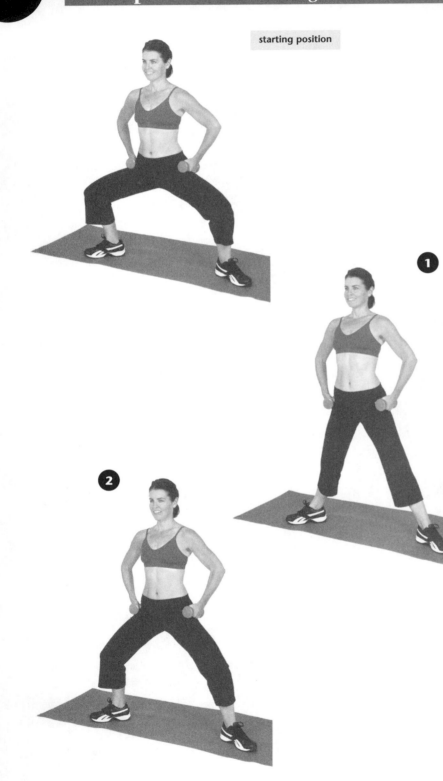

starting position

STARTING POSITION: Plant your feet at least three feet wide in a turned-out stance, with both knees bent. Holding a weight in each hand, perch one weight on top of each thigh. **INHALE** to begin.

1 **EXHALE** and straighten your knees. Try to move through your maximum range of motion and keep your shoulders directly above your hips, as if sliding up and down an invisible wall.

2 **INHALE** and return to the starting position.

MODIFICATION
Make the movement smaller by bending the knees less.

starting position

STARTING POSITION: Plant your feet at least three feet apart in a turned-out stance. Bend both knees and lift both heels off the floor—they should stay off the floor throughout the exercise. Holding a weight in each hand, perch a weight on top of each thigh. **INHALE** to begin.

1 **EXHALE** and straighten your knees.

2 **INHALE** and return to the starting position.

MODIFICATION

Pick up only one heel at a time and alternate from heel to heel. Your balance will be easier to maintain.

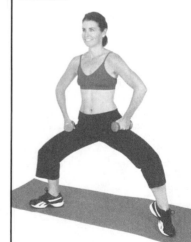

standing leg extension back

target: glutes

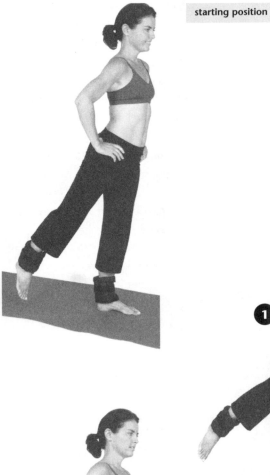

starting position

①

②

STARTING POSITION: Strap an ankle weight onto each ankle. Balance on your left leg and extend your right leg straight back, lifting it up anywhere from 3 to 6 inches off the ground. Pretend as if you have no knee on the raised leg for this exercise. Point your toe, too, if you can. **INHALE** to begin.

1 **EXHALE** and press your left leg farther back repeatedly in a pulsing manner. Be sure to really feel the lift of your butt cheek!

2 When you are done with your reps, switch sides.

MODIFICATION

If you have trouble balancing, hold onto a wall or the back of a chair for support. If the challenge is too intense, omit the weights altogether.

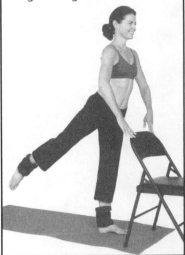

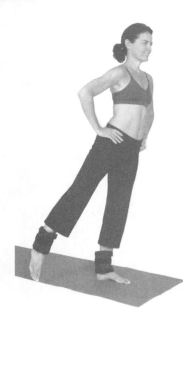

starting position

STARTING POSITION: Strap an ankle weight onto each ankle. Balance on your right leg and extend the left leg straight back 1 to 3 inches off the ground. Pretend as if you have no knee on the raised leg for this exercise.

1 With your left leg, trace a clockwise circle the size of a standard Frisbee to the rear of your body.

2 Now trace a counterclockwise circle.

3 When you are done with your reps, step your foot down and switch sides.

MODIFICATION

If you have trouble balancing, hold onto a wall or the back of a chair for support. If the challenge is too intense, omit the weights altogether.

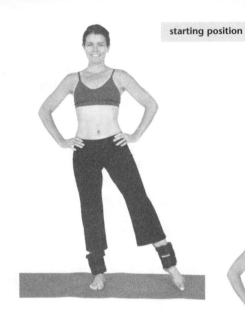

starting position

STARTING POSITION: Strap an ankle weight onto each ankle. Balance on your right leg and extend your left leg out to the side and up so that it's just grazing the floor. Point your toes, if possible. Pretend as if you have no knee on the extended leg. **INHALE** to begin.

1 **EXHALE** and press your left leg up a bit higher and repeatedly pulse upward.

2 When you're done with your reps, step down and switch sides.

MODIFICATION

If you have trouble balancing, hold onto a wall or the back of a chair for support. If the challenge is too intense, omit the weights altogether.

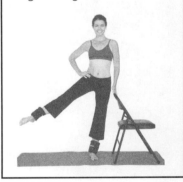

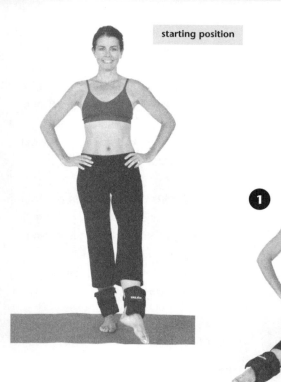

starting position

STARTING POSITION: Strap an ankle weight onto each ankle. Balance on your right leg and lift the left leg a few inches off the ground in front of your body. **INHALE** to begin.

1 **EXHALE** and press your left leg higher across your body, as if you were kicking a soccer ball. Repeatedly pulse it up and across.

2 When you're done with your reps, step down and switch sides.

1

2

MODIFICATION

If you have trouble balancing, hold onto a wall or the back of a chair for support. If the challenge is too intense, omit the weights altogether.

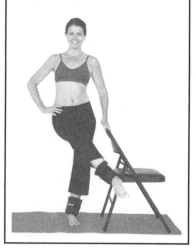

calf raise parallel

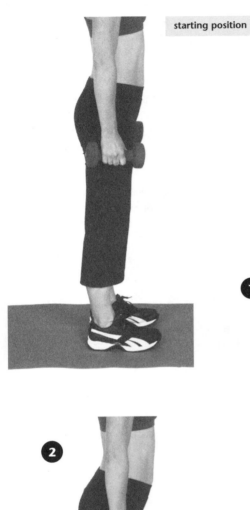

starting position

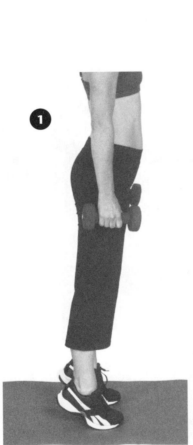

1

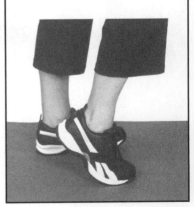

2

STARTING POSITION: Stand with your feet about 6 inches apart and your toes pointing forward. It's important to keep your knees straight and stiff but not locked. Hold a weight in each hand by your sides. **INHALE** to begin.

1 **EXHALE** and rise up onto the balls of both feet, moving only at the ankles. Squeeze your calf muscles. Take your time and aim for the fullest range of motion possible.

2 **INHALE** and return to the starting position.

MODIFICATION

Perform the exercise one leg at a time.

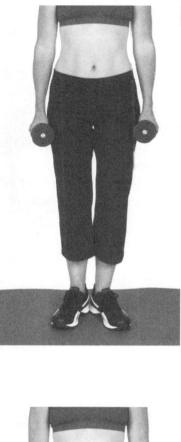

starting position

STARTING POSITION: Stand with your feet in a moderate turn-out with your heels together. Keep your entire body upright and maintain proper posture by stabilizing your core muscles. Hold a weight in each hand at your sides. **INHALE** to begin.

1 **EXHALE** and rise up onto the balls of both feet, moving only at the ankles. Squeeze your calf muscles. Take your time and aim for the fullest range of motion possible.

2 **INHALE** and return to the starting position.

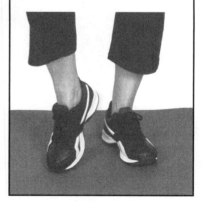

MODIFICATION

Perform the exercise one leg at a time.

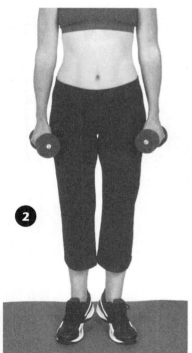

starting position

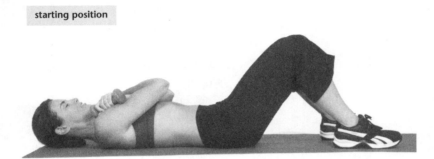

STARTING POSITION: Lie on your back with both knees bent. Take one weight in each hand and crisscross your forearms over your chest. Bring your chin toward your chest. **INHALE** to begin.

1 **EXHALE** and lift your shoulders completely off the mat, crunching your abdominal muscles.

2 **INHALE** and return the upper back to the floor.

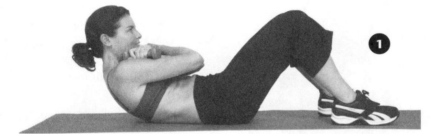

1

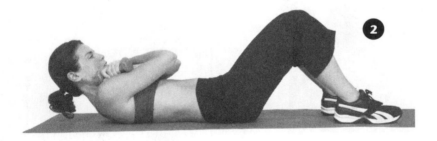

2

starting position

STARTING POSITION: Lie on your back with both knees bent and dropped to the right. Bring your right hand behind your head, opening your chest to the ceiling. Hold both weights in your left hand and place your left hand on the left side of your waist. **INHALE** to begin.

1 **EXHALE** and lift your shoulders completely off the mat, crunching the oblique muscles. Feel as though your goal is to squeeze the rib cage down toward the hip bone.

2 **INHALE** and return to the starting position. Once you've done all your reps, repeat on the other side.

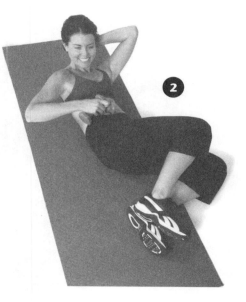

starting position

STARTING POSITION: Lie on your back with your legs straight up toward the ceiling, forming a 90-degree "L" with your body. Hold a weight on each side of your body for balance. **INHALE** to begin.

1 **EXHALE** and lift your hips up off the mat approximately 3 to 6 inches.

2 **INHALE** and lower your hips back to the starting position.

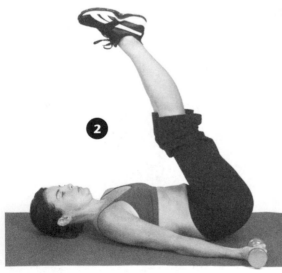

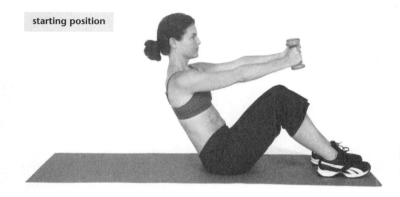

starting position

1

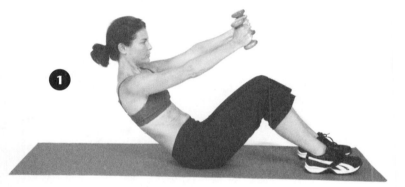

2

3

STARTING POSITION: Hold one weight in each hand and sit with your knees bent in front of you, leaning back slightly to form a "V" with your thighs and torso. **INHALE** to begin.

1 **EXHALE** and round your back toward the mat, articulating the spine one vertebra at a time, keeping the weights at arm's length in front of your chest.

2 Once your body makes full contact with the mat, open your arms wide like airplane wings and **INHALE**.

3 **EXHALE** and roll back up. When you reach the top, extend your arms overhead to challenge your upper back muscles.

starting position

STARTING POSITION: Lie on your back with the soles of your feet touching and your knees apart, in the shape of a diamond. Cross your arms over your chest, holding the weights comfortably upon each shoulder. **INHALE** to begin.

1 **EXHALE** and curl your head, neck and shoulders off the mat.

2 **INHALE** and return to the mat with control.

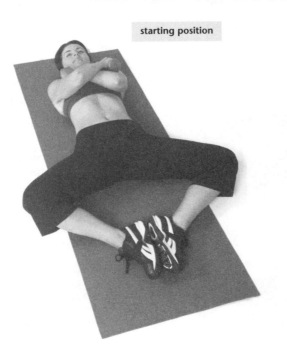

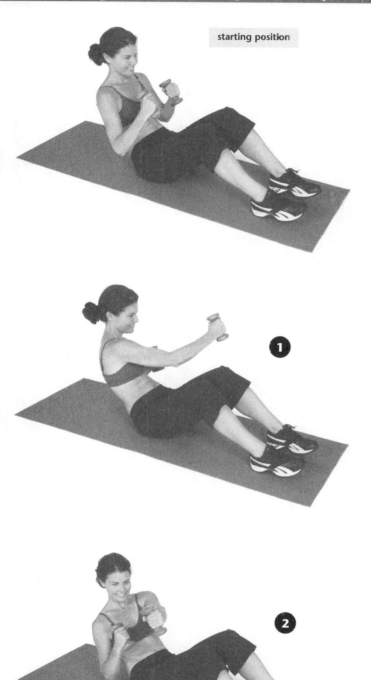

starting position

1

2

STARTING POSITION: Holding one weight in each hand, sit in a reclined position, as if you're in a bucket seat. Keep your knees bent and both feet firmly on the floor. Keep your shoulders down—shrugging will cause undesirable neck tension. **INHALE** to begin.

1 Like a boxer, **EXHALE** and punch your right arm across your body, extending through the elbow and twisting your torso to the left.

2 **INHALE** to return to center, then **EXHALE** as you punch your left arm across your body, extending through the elbow and twisting your torso to the other side. Repeat, alternating right and left, in a smooth, rhythmic pace.

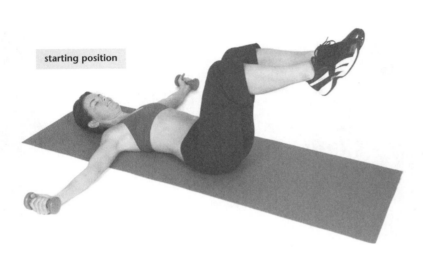

starting position

STARTING POSITION: Lie on your back with your arms extended out to the side like airplane wings, holding a weight in each hand with the palms facing up. Bring both knees up so that they stack over your hips. Your shins are parallel to the floor in a "table top" position. Relax your head, neck and shoulders. Both shoulders should remain on the mat throughout the exercise.

1 **INHALE** and, without disturbing your upper body, drop both knees to the right.

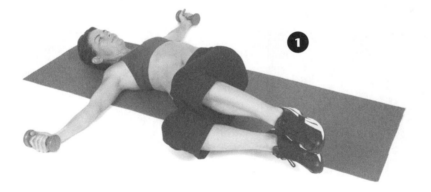

1

2 **EXHALE** and squeeze the knees back to the starting position.

3 **INHALE** and drop your knees to the left.

Aim for a total of 20 reps, alternating right and left.

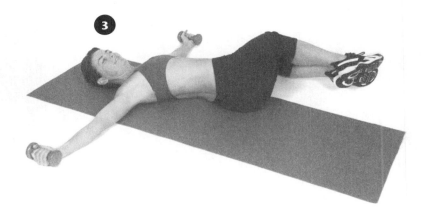

MODIFICATION

To increase your core's workload, strap an ankle weight to each ankle.

seated rowing
target: obliques/lower back/abs

starting position

STARTING POSITION: Combine both weights into both hands and sit in a reclined position, as if you're in a bucket seat. Your knees should be bent with both feet on the floor. Be sure to keep your shoulders down—shrugging will cause undesirable neck tension. **INHALE** to begin.

1 As if you were rowing a canoe, **EXHALE** and twist your body to the right as if paddling with the weights.

2 **INHALE** then **EXHALE** again and "paddle" to the left. Keep the movement smooth and fluid, alternating at a nice even pace.

starting position

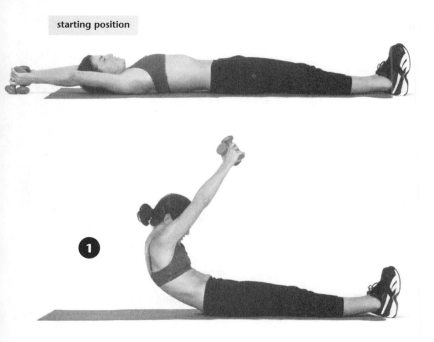

1

2

3

This exercise has a big range of motion and requires a lot of control.

STARTING POSITION: Lie on the floor with your legs straight and arms extended overhead. Hold a weight in each hand. **INHALE** to begin.

1 **EXHALE** and, keeping your upper arms close to your ears, crunch your abdominal muscles, curl your chin toward your chest, and slowly roll up. Keep your legs on the ground at all times.

2 At the top, **INHALE** and stretch your body over your legs.

3 **EXHALE** and return to the starting position, inhaling to reach your arms overhead.

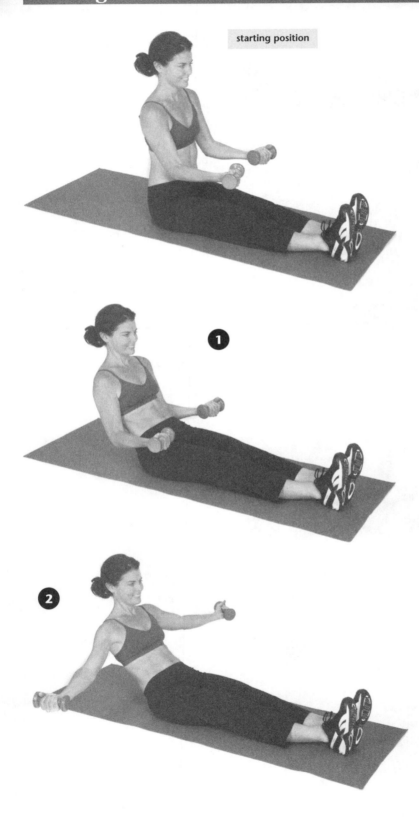

starting position

This move can also be performed without weights.

STARTING POSITION: Holding a weight in each hand, palms up, sit with your legs straight in front of you. Keep your elbows close to your sides and activate your core muscles. **INHALE** to begin.

1 **EXHALE** and, keeping your legs on the ground, roll back, as if getting into a bucket seat.

2 Using the same **EXHALE**, sweep your arms out to the side with control, moving your elbows away from your waist.

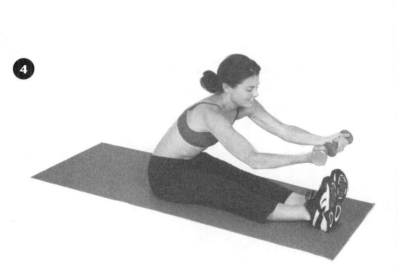

3 In one smooth but energized movement, **INHALE** and lengthen your spine upward and press your arms up.

4 **EXHALE** and, with control, roll your body forward, reaching the weights toward your toes.

MODIFICATION

To lessen the intensity on your lower back, bend your knees and plant your feet on the ground.

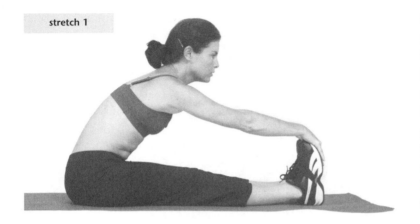

stretch 1

STRETCH 1: Sit on the floor with your legs extended straight in front of you. Inhale and extend both arms up overhead. Exhale and lean forward, draping your torso over your legs. If possible, grab onto your feet or shins and pull your body down slightly, accentuating the stretch. Stretch both legs simultaneously. Hold for 30–60 seconds.

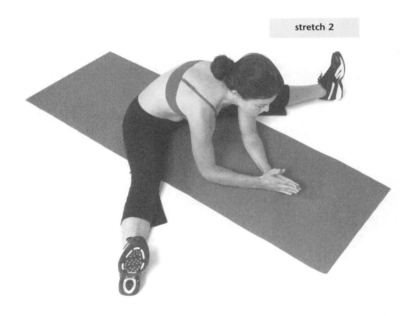

stretch 2

STRETCH 2: Sit on the floor and split your legs wide apart. Inhale and extend both arms up overhead. Exhale and lean forward, placing your hands or forearms on the floor or your legs. Hold for 30–60 seconds.

STRETCH 3: From Stretch 2, walk your hands to one side and drape your torso over that leg. After 30–60 seconds, slowly walk your body to the other side.

stretch 3

stretch 1

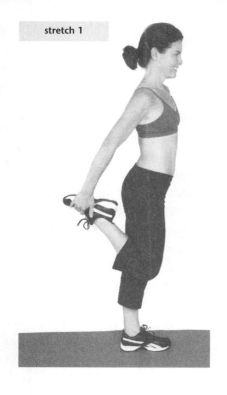

STRETCH 1: Stand with both feet together, then bring one heel to your butt. Grasp your foot with the same-side hand and try to keep your knees together. Hold for 30–60 seconds then switch sides. If balance is an issue, hold on to a chair or wall for support.

STRETCH 2: Sit on the floor with your legs slightly apart. Gently fold your left foot by your left hip. If your knee hurts, slowly release out of the pose and skip this stretch. If your knee feels fine, slowly lean back on your elbows, feeling the stretch in the front of your thigh. Hold for 30–60 seconds then switch sides. For a more intense stretch, you can also lie flat on the floor—but only if it doesn't hurt your knee.

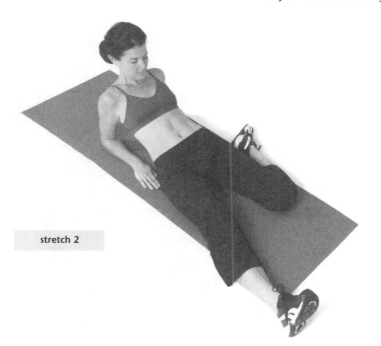

stretch 2

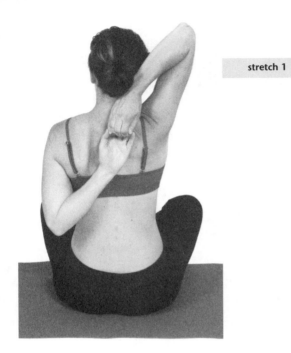

stretch 1

This can be done while sitting or standing.

STRETCH 1: Raise your right arm over your head and bend your elbow so that your right hand is behind your head. With your left hand, grasp the fingers of your right hand. (The elbow should point straight up.) Hold this position for 30–60 seconds then repeat the process with your left arm.

STRETCH 2: If you cannot grasp your fingers behind your back, simply apply pressure to the elevated elbow with your free hand.

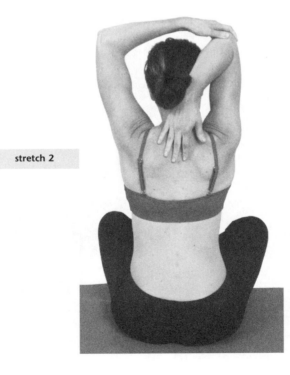

stretch 2

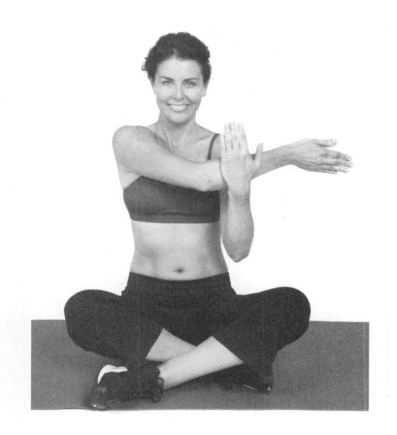

This can be done while standing or sitting.

Reach your right arm across your torso. Apply a bit of pressure with your left hand until you feel a stretch. Hold for 30–60 seconds then repeat the process with your left arm.

stretches
shoulder loop

1 Begin by shrugging your shoulders up toward your ears.

2 Now pull them straight back. Your shoulders will then, quite naturally, "drop," sliding down your back, seemingly lengthening your neck.

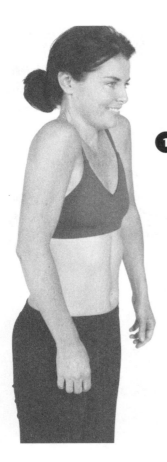

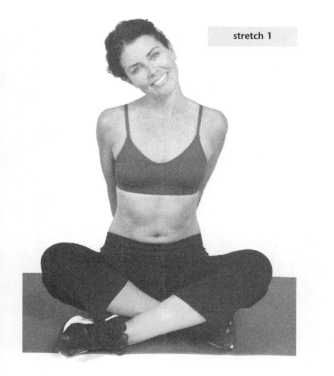

stretch 1

This can be done while standing or sitting.

STRETCH 1: Interlace your hands loosely behind your back and drop your right ear toward your right shoulder. Hold for 30–60 seconds then repeat the process on the other side.

STRETCH 2: Interlace your hands loosely behind your back and look to your left. Hold for 30–60 seconds then repeat the process on the other side.

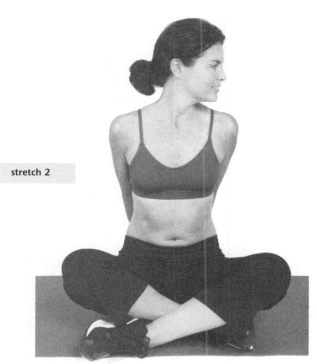

stretch 2

This can be done while standing or sitting. Here, we use the weight of the head to get a good stretch in the neck.

1 Gently and slowly relax your neck back.

2 Bring the chin down toward the chest.

3 Slowly roll your left ear toward your left shoulder, then roll your chin back down toward the chest before rolling your right ear toward your right shoulder.

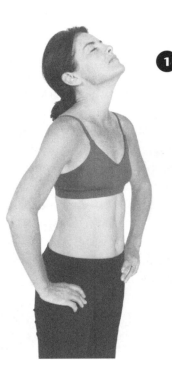

1

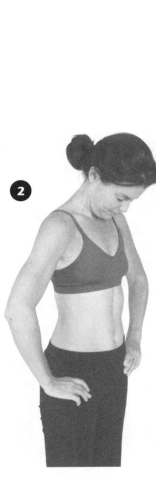

2

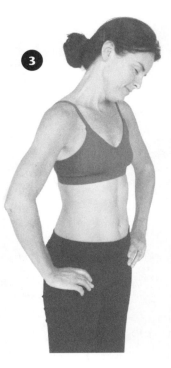

3

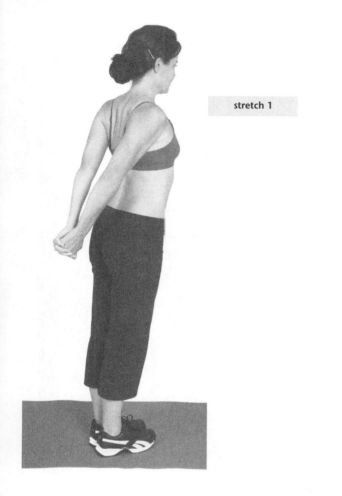

stretch 1

STRETCH 1: From a standing position, clasp your hands behind your back. Try to straighten your elbows and lift your arms up and away from your body. Hold for 30–60 seconds.

STRETCH 2: Place your hands on the back of a chair, then slowly walk your feet backward until your torso is parallel to the floor. Feel your chest open and stretch. Hold for 30–60 seconds.

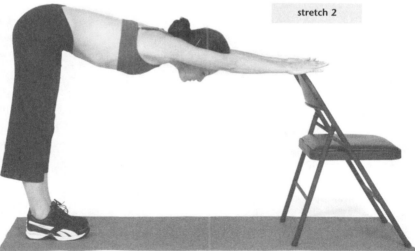

stretch 2

index

other books by ulysses press

ASHTANGA YOGA FOR WOMEN: INVIGORATING MIND, BODY AND SPIRIT WITH POWER YOGA
Sally Griffyn & Michaela Clarke, $17.95

Presents the exciting and empowering practice of power yoga in a balanced fashion that addresses the specific needs of female practitioners.

BALLET-FIT WORKOUT: DEVELOP STRENGTH, CONTROL, FLEXIBILITY & GRACE
Megan Connelly, Paula Baird-Colt & David McAllister, $16.95

Optimal health is the focus throughout *Ballet-Fit Workout*, and the authors show how classic dance training not only reshapes the body but also teaches mental focus and leads to a calm, refreshed mind.

BELLY DANCING FOR FITNESS: THE ULTIMATE DANCE WORKOUT THAT UNLEASHES YOUR CREATIVE SPIRIT
Tamalyn Dallal with Richard Harris, $14.95

A healthy aerobic workout that adds dancing, exotic music, the twirl of silk and the rhythmic clanging of finger cymbals.

ELLIE HERMAN'S PILATES WORKBOOK ON THE BALL: ILLUSTRATED STEP-BY-STEP GUIDE
Ellie Herman, $13.95

Combines the powerful slimming and shaping effects of Pilates with the low-impact, high-intensity workout of the ball.

FORZA: THE SAMURAI SWORD WORKOUT
Ilaria Montagnani, $14.95

Transforms sword-fighting techniques into a program that combines the excitement of sword play with a heart-pumping, full-body workout.

THE MARTIAL ARTIST'S BOOK OF YOGA: IMPROVE FLEXIBILITY, BALANCE AND STRENGTH FOR HIGHER KICKS, FASTER STRIKES, SMOOTHER THROWS, SAFER FALLS AND STRONGER STANCES
Lily Chou with Kathe Rothacher, $14.95

A great training supplement for martial artists, this book clearly illustrates how specific yoga poses can directly improve one's martial arts abilities.

POSTURE POWER FOR WOMEN: SIMPLE STEPS AND QUICK EXERCISES THAT TRANSFORM YOUR APPEARANCE AND IMPROVE YOUR HEALTH
Carol Armitage with Mike Bebb, $13.95

Helping women improve their lives by fixing their posture, *Posture Power for Women* reveals how better posture strengthens, energizes and revitalizes the body.

SEXY YOGA: 40 POSES FOR MIND-BLOWING SEX & GREATER INTIMACY
Ellen Barrett, $14.95

Sexy Yoga offers the modern yoga student a specific program designed to transform and heighten sexual pleasure and lovemaking.

ULTIMATE CORE BALL WORKOUT: STRENGTHENING AND SCULPTING EXERCISES WITH OVER 200 STEP-BY-STEP PHOTOS
Jeanine Detz, $14.95

Maximizes today's hottest area of fitness—core training—by tapping the power of the exercise ball with these strengthening and sculpting exercises.

WEIGHTS ON THE BALL WORKBOOK: STEP-BY-STEP GUIDE WITH OVER 350 PHOTOS
Steven Stiefel, $14.95

With exercises suited for all skill levels, *Weights on the Ball Workbook* shows how to simultaneously use weights and the exercise ball for the ultimate total-body workout.

WEIGHT-BEARING WORKOUTS FOR WOMEN: EXERCISES FOR SCULPTING, STRENGTHENING & TONING
Yolande Green, $12.95

Weight training is the fastest, most effective way to lose fat, improve muscle tone and strengthen bones. This workbook shows just how easy it is for women at any age to get started with weights.

WORKOUTS FROM BOXING'S GREATEST CHAMPS
Gary Todd, $14.95

Features dramatic photos, workout secrets and behind-the-scenes details of Muhammad Ali, Roy Jones, Jr., Fernando Vargas and other legends.

YOGA IN FOCUS: POSTURES, SEQUENCES AND MEDITATIONS
Jessie Chapman   photographs by Dhyan, $14.95

A beautiful celebration of yoga that's both useful for learning the techniques and inspiring in its artistic approach to presenting the body in yoga positions.

To order these books call 800-377-2542 or 510-601-8301, fax 510-601-8307, e-mail ulysses@ulyssespress.com, or write to Ulysses Press, P.O. Box 3440, Berkeley, CA 94703. All retail orders are shipped free of charge. California residents must include sales tax. Allow two to three weeks for delivery.

about the author

ELLEN BARRETT, the author of *Sexy Yoga* (Ulysses Press), holds a master's degree in education along with multiple certifications in Pilates, yoga, personal training and group exercise. She's been hailed as a pioneer—helping people conquer new frontiers—and has earned a stellar reputation in the fitness industry. A celebrity trainer and a star in many exercise videos, including *Crunch: Super Slim Down* (Anchor Bay Entertainment, 2006), she personifies the new age of fitness, where the mind, body and spirit converge for more intelligent, efficient workouts—like those showcased in this book. Ellen lives in New Haven, Connecticut, where she owns THE STUDIO by Ellen Barrett, a fusion fitness utopia just for women. For more information about Ellen, please visit www.EllenBarrett.com.